A Bend in the Road

A Year's Journey Through Breast Cancer

A Bend in the Road

A Year's Journey Through Breast Cancer

by Karen Kelly Boyce

KFR
Communications, LLC

A Bend in the Road: A Year's Journey Through Breast Cancer

Published by: KFR Communications, LLC
             148 Hawkin Rd
             New Egypt, NJ 08533

Publisher's Note: The author and publisher have taken care in preparation of this book but make no expressed or implied warranty of any kind and assume no responsibility for errors or omissions. No liability is assumed for incidental or consequential damages in connection with or arising out of the use of the information contained herein.

ISBN-10: 0-6920-0925-6
ISBN-13: 978-0-692-00925-3

Printed in the United States of America

www.kfrcommunications.com

Dedication

This work is dedicated to the physicians of The Cancer Institute of New Jersey and Robert Wood Johnson University Hospital, especially Dr. Thomas Kearney & Dr. Antoinette Tan.

The proceeds of this work will be evenly donated to both the research of oncology by Dr. Antoinette Tan & the fellowship cost of those who study surgery under Dr. Thomas Kearney.

I would also like to thank all of those who prayed for me during my fight with cancer.

I'd also like to remember Carol Serrel - who lost her valiant fight with cancer - but in honor of her and many others, the fight to save lives continues.

Most of all, I would like to give thanks to the God of Healing who was ever with me in my time of need.

Contents

Introduction

I have always loved paintings and photos displaying roads - roads that wind through the woods, paths leading along flowing rivers or shimmering lakes. I love Thomas Kincaid's work because he often paints a road that leads to a warmly lit cottage or a beckoning chapel.

While in Ireland years ago, I purchased an oil painting to commemorate the town Bantry Bay. My great-grandfather was born in Bantry Bay. It presented a young Shepherd guiding his flock of sheep along a dirt road lined with the emerald green grass and the rocky fences of the magical island. It is entitled, *The Road to Bantry Bay*.

It reminded me of the 23rd Psalm. We are on a road. I like to think that our Shepherd, the Good Shepherd, is guiding our steps. I know He guides mine.

We are all on a unique and strange journey; a journey back to the God who created us. When we are young, and we look ahead, the road seems so long. We think we have all the time in the world. Yet because we have so much we want to accomplish we rush down the road, anxious to see what's ahead of us. When we are toddlers, we can't wait for kindergarten. When on a tricycle, we long for that two-wheeler. In elementary school, we cannot wait until high school.

We are always pushing ahead, anxious to grow up and enter the next stage of life. We want our independence and we can't be stopped as we rush down the road. We hurry to college or a job. We set our sights on marriage, then children. We don't have time to wait. We are on a journey and we feel we have to quicken our pace to get everything done. Often we hurry so hastily that we fail to take the time to look around.

We don't look at the places and people who surround us each day, never taking the time to look to the side, to see the time and the place of our journey. We seldom wonder why we were born in this country, during this precise century. Why weren't we born in Africa, why not in Europe or South America? There must be a reason. There must be a explanation why we weren't born during the French Revolution or the Middle Ages, or even during the Dark Ages? No, we are too busy rushing along the road to consider what it is that we need to contribute to our age.

Have you ever taken the time to look at the people who travel with you, the sojourners who share your road? In childhood, we gravitate to those who skip at the same beat, locking arms; we swear lifelong allegiance as we swap blood oaths to unending friendship. However, something seems to happen when we journey ahead. Some of those friends, who walked with us, rush ahead or seem to fall behind. As our journey continues, we notice that different companions wander with us for short times. If we are blessed, some of those companions will keep us company for a long time.

As a teenager, I loved the poem by Robert Frost, *The Road Not Taken*. It inspired me although I never had the courage it portrayed. I thought Robert Frost understood the way of life. Now I realize he may have been wrong. We don't have to look for the road not traveled, for whatever way we go is unique. No one has ever walked the road we take and no one in the future ever will. We alone, see the times and places we have seen. We alone meet the wonderful people we encounter along the way. No one else can have the exact same adventures, experiences, or loves.

We meet such diverse and unique characters to share our journey. Make no mistake; however, no matter how many friends share our walk, this is a personal journey. While the road that leads home might be familiar to all of us, each person walks alone. Young, we think the road is straight. But it never is.

We all reach a bend in the road, a path that takes us off the main thoroughfare, which separates us from the well-worn way. We are all led to the bend in the road, which stops our steady march forward. We are seldom ready for it. For each of us the bend comes at a different time in our lives. For me, the separate path was breast cancer. For you, it could be an illness or a divorce. For many, it has been the death of someone close. It can even be a financial crisis. Only one thing is sure. We all come to a bend in the road. It leads us to a side path on our journey. This book is the story of my journey.

I wasn't prepared for the side path. My life was going full steam ahead. My children had grown and started their own travels. I was retired from nursing. Finally, I could pursue a dream - a dream of being a writer. I poured my soul out on paper. A novel finished. The dream of being published came true. Holding my first novel in my hands gave me a sense of a deeper meaning to my life. Then, just as I was about to share my dream, I hit a bend in the road - breast cancer. It meant a year on a separate path. When I entered the path, I didn't know where it would lead. Would it loop around, leading back to the road of my life? I wasn't sure, and could only take one step after another on the uneven trail.

Looking around, the vegetation seemed dense. Looking back, I noticed that some of my favorite companions were continuing on the main road. They were leaving me to travel alone, afraid of losing time. Nevertheless, I found others, some taking a similar side trail. Stricken with cancer; they too, walked the unfamiliar track. I noticed others. On the main road, they were just acquaintances but they slowed a little to encourage me along the side path. Companions who stopped a while, painting hope with kind words and prayers. They suddenly became friends.

When I started this book, I was sure it would be a comedy. Cancer can be so depressing. I wanted to take a different view. So many experiences have been downright funny. I wanted to share those, to make you laugh. A strange thing happened, however, when

I started to write my great comedy. I couldn't do it. I struggled for weeks - revamping this paragraph, restructuring that sentence - nothing seemed to help.

Finally, I stopped to pray about it. My heart spoke truth. Nothing but the whole truth would do. My journey through breast cancer was both joyful, and sad. I laughed and I cried. I lost faith and yet clung to hope. This was the whole truth, and nothing but the whole truth was worth telling. Therefore, yes, I hope to make you laugh. God knows I did. However, I also hope make you cry, pray, and, learn something to prepare you for when you hit your bend in the road. So, link arms with me for a short time. Slow down and walk a little way with me.

Foreword

I was very touched when I was asked to write the foreword for this book. As a physician who works in an academic medical center and specializes in the treatment of breast cancer, it is an uncommon request, but a fitting one in this specific instance. Concern about breast cancer is likely to cross every woman's mind at some point in her life. We are always hearing how prevalent breast cancer is. Every woman who faces this diagnosis has her own personal journey to share. This one is no exception.

I became a breast medical oncologist for several reasons: the opportunity to form life-long relationships with patients, the chance to work with a multidisciplinary team of experts, and the access to clinical research. Patients with breast cancer go through a variety of emotions during their care: anxiety at initial diagnosis, trepidation of surgery, the fear of unknown side effects from chemotherapy, endocrine and/or targeted therapy, the relief at the completion of therapy, and ambivalence during the transition from active treatment to follow-up. I admire every patient's unique way of coping with her situation. The best breast cancer care requires close collaboration between the medical oncologist, surgeon, radiologist, pathologist, radiation oncologist, nurse, social worker, and research staff. This team approach is so important for the successful delivery of care. On a personal level, the intellectual stimulation and camaraderie that comes with being part of a multidisciplinary team is a satisfying day-to-day experience.

The research aspect of my career is an important one I would like to share. As a fourth-year medical student, I spent five weeks on the medical oncology service at the National Cancer Institute. I followed several patients with a variety of cancers through their course on different clinical trials. I shared their joy over the success of treatments and their disappointment when the therapies were not so effective. The rotation also introduced me to the rigors of a clinical research study. It was then that I realized where I could have an impact. Motivated to learn more about oncology and the field of clinical research, I completed my residency training in internal medicine and returned to the National Cancer Institute for a fellowship in medical oncology. During the first year of my oncology fellowship, I developed more of an understanding of the conduct of clinical trials as I enrolled patients onto protocols of investigational treatments and cared for them firsthand. I was fortunate to obtain formal training in clinical trial design and statistics and eventually a master's degree in clinical research.

In 2003, I began working at the Cancer Institute of New Jersey to develop, implement and conduct clinical trials in breast cancer with a focus on translating basic science discoveries to the clinic. It has been and continues to be a very rewarding experience. I remain committed to designing trials that answer important research questions that will lead to the development of new anti-cancer drugs and therapies for patients with breast cancer. I am moved that the proceeds from this book will be donated for this research.

Breast cancer is a complex disease. Research discoveries are advancing rapidly due to our increased understanding of molecular biology. The collaborative efforts of basic scientists, clinical researchers, and patients who participate on trials are a major way we can continue to provide state-of-the-art treatment. The future holds great promise for further breakthroughs. I am humbled by my patients' efforts to live and share their journey.

Antoinette R. Tan, MD, MHSc
Medical Oncologist
The Cancer Institute of New Jersey
Robert Wood Johnson Medical School
University of Medicine and Dentistry of New Jersey

Doctors

I was standing in the checkout line at the supermarket, when I heard the fuss. There was no choice; I had to turn around and find out what the crowd was gathering to see.

Somehow, I knew it would involve my four-year-old son. There he was, so cute with his Buster Brown haircut and his blue and orange Yankee jacket. So cute...with his hand stuck up the gumball machine. A growing number of onlookers encircled him, but at the center of the crowd were the men who were clearly in charge of the situation. The store manager and two pimple-faced teenagers in white aprons were rubbing their chins and assessing the situation.

The female cashier called the police for help. When the squad car arrived with lights flashing, I stood with the rest of the crowd; sure that the situation was well in hand. The police officer used all the weight of his authority to push the crowd back and give my immobile son some room.

The ambulance arrived and two paramedics carrying toolboxes stepped into the store. The crowd parted, letting the men assess the situation. My son remained stuck amongst the gumballs; his hand not visible among the enticing treats. The store manager, two store clerks, one police officer, and two paramedics stood looking at the gumball machine, as if waiting for something to happen.

The fire truck, with sirens blaring, pulled in front of the store. Firefighters entered, with heavy boots beneath the official pants. The lights of the fire engine whirled in mesmerizing colors through the window. My son smiled, exposing his dimples.

Turning to me in excitement he shouted, "Mommy, look at the fire engine! Could I have a ride?"

Before my son spoke and identified me as his mother, I had tried to melt into the on-looking crowd. The store manager looked up and with his eyes glaring, memorized my face, perhaps for a future poster. I imagined the poster hanging on the large entrance door: Do not admit this woman - bad mother.

With reddened face, I smiled and nodded at the professionals, giving them permission to correct the situation now seen as my fault. One of the firefighters removed the red ceramic gumball top and lifted the glass bowl holding the gumballs. The gumballs fell through the opening in the bottom and hit the tiled floor. Like marbles they rolled, past the cash registers and down the aisles.

My son remained standing, with his fisted hand the only object resting on the base of the gumball machine.

One of the fire fighters examined the opening and said, "I think if we take a screwdriver and remove the facing, we'll be able to pull his hand through."

One of the paramedics spoke up, "Perhaps I should cover his hand with some lubricant."

The men pondered the suggestions as the cashier who had called for help walked up to my prodigy.

Looking at him with eyes full of experience she said "Let go of the gumball, son."

He did. I watched as the single gumball fell to the floor and rolled and down the aisle. With his hand relaxed, my son pulled it out of the gumball machine on his own.

I walked up to him and took his chin in my hand, "Why didn't you just let go of the gumball right away?"

His eyes welled with tears, and he sobbed, "Caaause...I got a red one!"

The paramedic examined his perfect hand, as the manager and

store clerks started sweeping up the gumballs. Turning to me he said, "Do you want us to take him to the emergency room for an x-ray?"

"No," I replied as I started to leave, lugging my one bag of groceries and my son. "I'll take him right over to my doctor." I was anxious to make my escape, knowing I would be shopping at the supermarket across town for the next few months.

My doctor had taken care of my family for years. He was an old man with thick, white hair and a creased face. It was a kind face with merry eyes. The Irish have a saying: "In the end everyone ends up with the face they earn." My doctor had earned his loving countenance.

I could call him whenever I needed him. His receptionist, trained from 30 years of working for him, always said, "Come over to the office, but you might have to wait for a short while."

This day was no exception; 'waiting for short while' was an understatement. I waited for hours because most of the people in the waiting room had called that day in crisis. No one had a prearranged appointment. The doctor didn't operate that way. Waiting was the price paid for seeing him on the day I needed him. I knew enough to bring a good book to read.

After the doctor stopped laughing, he declared my son in perfect health. We were on our way home with a lollipop and a fond farewell. He was the right kind of doctor for me because I was a 'crisis management' type of girl. I didn't see the point of wasting my time seeing a doctor when I felt fine. Would you bring your car to the garage if it were running great? Would you run to the supermarket if your pantry were full? I hated to waste time. Wasting a few hours in the waiting room every few years was little price to pay for attention on demand.

Five years later, I was on my deck barbecuing. After flipping the burger, I turned to see a strange look on my daughter's face.

"What's the matter?" I asked.

"I dond knowah. My towong ist too bick" she struggled to reply.

I had never seen anything like it. Her swollen tongue was a

blueberry color. Of course, we were off to the doctor.

Looking at the blue tongue, he seemed amazed. "I've never seen a tongue that color. Did she eat anything strange?"

He didn't do tests. He took the time to stop and ask some questions. Had she done anything strange? No. Had any strange animal been around? No. Had I noticed anything strange in her environment? A vague memory hit me. That morning, as I was cutting, forming, and marinating the meat for the barbecue, I remember seeing an unusual sight through the kitchen window.

My husband was on a mission. The previous day, a wasp stung him, and all morning he had been mumbling about the fate of any bug that had the nerve to come near him. I paid little attention as he visited the giant depot store. He was busy with his plans for revenge. I remember thinking how severe payback had become, when I saw he had a respirator on and a sprayer attached to our hose. Poison was my husband's choice of retribution, and plenty of it. No bug had a chance. He sprayed the ground, the trees, the garage, and the deck. Then, he sprayed them all again.

Poisoning the environment was against my nature, but I knew better than to disturb a man on a mission. I continued my plans and left the man to find happiness in his own way. I never connected my daughter's blue tongue to my husband's settling of scores. The doctor did. My daughter was allergic to insecticide. Doc didn't need any test to make his diagnosis. He rarely ordered a test and if he did, it was just to confirm what he already knew.

He treated me with the same method. Most physicians insisted on time consuming and uncomfortable yearly tests. I was of the opinion that if it couldn't be done in the office - during one of my emergency visits - I didn't have time for it. Oh sure, my doctor would mention the tests and even strongly recommend them. We played a game. He would tell me to call and make an appointment. I would listen and nod. I would get the medical attention I needed at the time. Not surprisingly, he would never receive a call from me until the next medical crisis occurred.

He never harassed me about my lifestyle or my extra weight. He gave me antibiotics for ear infections and gave the kids their shots. To my way of thinking, he was a superlative doctor. I would have gladly kept him as my physician for the rest of my life.

Unfortunately, all good things end. My husband's union changed their insurance coverage and my doctor was no longer an option. The search began. I started to call physicians in a very scientific manner. A manner reflecting the education I acquired as a working R.N.; I pulled out the yellow pages and made my calls based on how near the doctor was to my home. My main inquiry was, "Do you accept this insurance?"

Within an hour, I had an appointment with a new doctor. Even better, the doctor was in the same town, and could see me the next day. It was great. It wasn't that I needed to see a physician. I didn't have a crisis at the time, but I knew I had to establish a relationship before I could see the doctor in an emergency.

Now my only concern was to pick out a book to bring with me to read in the waiting room. I thought I was set; not realizing my troubles were just beginning.

The waiting room was not crowded, that was a bad sign. Perhaps it was an off day. I filled out my life story on the clipboard papers the nurse handed me. The autobiography you had to write was the cost paid for being new. It didn't take me long; I only had a crisis management type of history. The efficient looking - and very dour nurse - led me to the examining room. Without cracking a smile, she weighed and measured me with scale and cuff.

Reaching into the cabinet, she handed me an extra large Johnny coat with ripped ties and announced, "Take everything off and put this on. The doctor will be here in a minute." Doing as she instructed, I pouted as I sat.

Casually, I asked, "This is my first visit. What is the doctor like?"

For the first time, the nurse smiled and answered as she exited the examination room, "Oh you'll like her. She's very nice."

'She', 'her' - I hadn't missed the words. Oh no, I thought, the doctor is a woman. Now, I know what you're thinking. No, I think woman doctors are just as smart and competent as their male counterparts are. I had only one problem with going to a female doctor. My feminine wiles wouldn't work on her.

I had always managed to avoid going for the routine tests my doctor wanted everyone to have each year. Oh, I'm sure you know them - Pap smears, EKG's, x-rays, mammograms. I hated tests and quite frankly just didn't have the inclination to waste my time in waiting rooms once a year. Besides, my medical philosophy had always been that if a doctor looks long enough, he is sure to find something wrong, something that would require you to slow down, lose weight, or just stop having fun.

Oh sure, I was a nurse and should have known better, but let me tell you, medical people are the worst patients. Probably because health professionals think they know everything. Some of the most disobedient patients I have ever handled were doctors and nurses. They never followed instructions, took their medicine, or listened to recommendations. Maybe they are difficult because they don't have the respect for medical personnel the public has. They have seen what happens to a patient who gets hooked on the endless wheel of medical visits.

Just when I thought things couldn't get any worse, they did. I was sitting on the paper-lined table in my Johnny coat with the broken ties, when the new doctor walked in. Oh God help me, she was young, and beautiful. She weighed about fifty pounds. Tossing her long blond hair, she glanced at me and with a look of distain, decided that I would have to change my lifestyle. With no introduction, and no chance to soften her up with a joke, she announced, "You've not been taking care of yourself, have you? Do you know that your weight is way out of line with the recommended weight for your height?"

It was my policy when people were rude or stupid enough to say something like, "Do you know that you're overweight?" or "Do you realize that being overweight is bad for you?" I would act shocked.

With my eyes widened and my mouth hanging open, I would answer, "You mean, you think I'm overweight?"

It usually left them speechless. I quickly assessed the situation here. This new doctor didn't look as if she had a sense of humor. She bustled around the room in her starched and ironed lab coat - size two - without cracking a smile.

She looked down my throat, in my ears, and in my eyes as I kept my silence. Pulling out my chart, she looked shocked, "When did you have your last Pap smear?" Now I hated to tell her, but I knew the exact year. My last Pap smear was taken during my postpartum visit after the birth of my son. The problem was that my son was about to graduate college.

I meekly whispered the lie, "I don't really remember."

Not about to let me off the hook, she asked another question, "When was your last mammogram?"

Now I knew that it was recommended that women get a mammogram once a year after the age of forty. What could I say; I never took the time to have one. I thought she might faint.

Leaving the office with two bandaged arms from the draconian bloodletting the doctor had insisted on; I could feel the gooey moisture from the EKG electrodes on my back. I unhappily carried a pamphlet describing a 1,200-calorie, low-fat diet in one hand and a prescription for a mammogram in the other. I approached the receptionist's desk. Would I really go for the mammogram? I tried to be philosophical. My new insurance covered a yearly mammogram.

The receptionist settled the question announcing, "The doctor wants to see you in a month, so you better have the mammogram right away. I'll make the appointment for you."

There was no escape. I decided that once I appeased the doc with one mammogram, I would probably be good for life.

Tests

The mammogram uses a special, low-dose x-ray machine to take pictures of both breasts. The results are recorded on x-ray film or directly onto a computer for a radiologist to examine.[1] There are two kinds of mammograms. The most common - the kind I had - is a film screen mammography. The breast is positioned and compressed between two plates and a camera takes two pictures of each breast from different angles. A radiologist will read the film. Sometimes your mammogram film can be read by a computer, which can find any area with extra thickness in the breast tissue. This is called CAD or computer-aided detection.

The second kind of mammogram is called digital mammography. In this mammography, the image is recorded directly into a computer so the radiologist can enlarge any suspicious area and take a closer look. This digital mammography is not available on a widespread basis but seems to be the wave of the future. It also enables the experts to manipulate the image on monitors and quickly send the image to other experts or physicians. The mammograms can be done at a hospital, or a clinic.

I drove past the clinic twice before I found it. By the time I did, I was 15 minutes late. It didn't matter. The office was packed with people. The clinic did all kinds of x-rays, ultrasounds, and scans. People waited with broken legs. Children with casts cried. I settled in the plastic chair with a resolve to wait patiently.

I thought my wait would be long, but a nurse came out from behind a door and called my name before I could even get bored.

The tall, thin nurse led me down a hallway, past various rooms. In those rooms, patients were being spun and bent in various strange positions as machines hummed and whirred around them. Nothing prepared me for the room I was to enter.

The room was dark and cool. The large machine took up half of the room. It reminded me of something I had seen years ago. In the 70s - while I was in college - we all went on a trip to see something called a 'thinking machine.' It was a large machine, which took up the whole wall of the lab. It lay flat against the long 20 foot wall, and looked like a curio cabinet. The front was covered in glass, and beneath that glass, large tapes whirled back and forth making a lot of noise. The professor announced that the machine was so intelligent that it could play and beat humans at the card game 21. A few of my classmates played against the machine and lost. The professor announced on the way back to the classroom that this machine was the future. He announced that he was going to invest some money in the research. I figured he was crazy. Who would ever find a use for something as stupid as this machine they called a computer?

The tall nurse was apparently the one who was going to administer the test. She looked down at me and said, "Strip to the waist. Have you ever had a mammogram before?"

Sheepishly, I answered, as I stripped, "No, this is my first."

The nurse turned on the machine and pushed a button to lower a tray. Squeezing, squeezing, the machine just keep squeezing. Just when I lost my breath from the tight spot that I found myself in, the nurse yelled, "Don't breathe now." She dove behind the shield, as the clicking of the machine confirmed that the image was being taken. Strange thoughts ran through my mind, as I remained stuck in the machine. What if there was a fire? Did I think this nurse would take the time to release me so I could escape? Wouldn't it be sad to die in such a strange position?

Finally released, the nurse studied the picture on a small TV-like screen.

"Looks good!" she announced. "Let's get a look at the other

breast and we can wrap this up."

The machine was set in place. Again, it was squeezing. Squeezing, and squeezing until I thought my eyes would pop out. The nurse went behind the shield and the machine clicked and whirled as the pictures were taken.

Staring at the same screen, the nurse's smile froze. Her eyes no longer smiled, "Hmm, I may need to take this one again. It's not as clear as I would like."

She moved the screen out of my view, but I had already seen it. The large white spot was hard to miss. I let her repeat the test. Maybe it was a bad image. No, the large white spot was still there. This time the nurse didn't hide it.

"See this spot." She pointed at the image. "This looks a little suspicious. I think we will have the doctor look at this. You know, if he thinks it's necessary, you may have to have a biopsy done. You can have it done here if you want."

I was glad to dress and find my way out of there. I didn't like the new sympathetic look in the nurse's eyes. I knew it! One test always led to another. I wasn't afraid that it might be cancer. Somewhere, in a magazine article, I had read that 80% of all abnormalities that mammograms found turned out to be harmless cysts. My girlfriend had cysts, and the doctor made her give up coffee.

Oh great, I thought. I loved my morning coffee. As if in defiance, I pulled through the Dunkin Donuts drive thru and ordered a large creamy carton of coffee. Somewhere on the drive home, I decided not to tell anyone. Why borrow trouble? It would probably be nothing. I didn't even want to think about giving up coffee.

Within a week, I was back at the clinic for a biopsy. There are four kinds of biopsies usually done to check lesions in the breast. One is an open excision biopsy. This procedure can be performed whether or not the breast mass is palpable and is usually performed under local anesthesia (i.e. the patient remains awake during the procedure). The area is numbed with a local anesthetic and a sedative is usually administered. A small incision of about one to two inches is made as close to the lump as possible. The surgeon removes a piece of tissue, or if it is small, the entire lump and the incision are sutured. The biopsy usually takes about an hour to perform.

If the lump cannot be felt, the procedure is slightly more involved and time consuming. Because it cannot be felt, it must be located by a process called needle localization. The patient goes to radiology and a mammogram is used to pinpoint the lump. A wire needle is inserted into the breast, marking the location of the lump. The wire is left inside the breast and taped to the skin, and the patient is taken to the operating room to have the biopsy.[2]

A needle biopsy is done if the lesion is palpable. It can be done in a doctor's office. The doctor uses a needle with a hollow center to obtain material for the lab to check. The needle is placed with the help of an x-ray or mammography. A collapsible hook at end of the needle keeps it in place until the surgery is done. This type of biopsy has the highest rate of 'false negatives', which is when a biopsy return is called normal even though cancer is actually present. This is because the needle doesn't always pick up the cancer cells in the lesion. However, results can be as quickly available in as little as 24 hours.

My doctor ordered a Stereo tactic needle biopsy - also called a core biopsy - to be done in the same clinic where I had the mammogram. This procedure is similar to fine needle aspiration, but the needle is larger, enabling a larger sample to be obtained. It is performed under local anesthesia and ultrasound or stereo tactic mammography is used if the lump cannot be felt. Three to six needle insertions are needed to obtain an adequate sample of tissue. A clicking sound may be heard as the samples are being taken and the patient may feel some pressure, but should not feel pain. The procedure takes a few minutes and no stitches are required. Core needle biopsy may provide a more accurate analysis and diagnosis than fine needle aspiration because tissue is removed, rather than just cells. This procedure is not accurate in patients with very small or hard lumps.[3]

The vacuum biopsy is another method. This method utilizes

a vacuum-like device to remove breast tissue. Local anesthesia is used and no incision is made. Stereo tactic mammography is used to guide a breast probe to the lesion. Computers pinpoint the mass and suction draws out the breast tissue. The needle is inserted once to obtain multiple samples. In some cases, the entire lesion may be removed.

Vacuum-assisted biopsy is safe, reliable, and valuable for patients who are not candidates for other minimally invasive biopsy techniques and those who wish to avoid surgical biopsy. The procedure should be performed by a highly skilled radiologist or surgeon who is experienced and familiar with this method.[4]

In this type of biopsy, multiple pieces of the affected area are removed. If the lesion can't be felt, the needle is guided with mammography or ultrasound.

I pulled into the clinic at 9:45am, not missing it on this morning. This time I had to report to the other side of the clinic, where I was introduced to the two women who would conduct the test.

The first woman was a doctor, the one who would do the biopsy. She seemed so young. Tall, thin, and dark-haired, she was sweet and kind. The nurse who was her assistant was more like me. Short and square, she seemed like a good egg, with a great sense of humor. I felt better just meeting them.

Unfortunately, they first had to repeat the mammogram. I didn't care; I was a pro by now. During this mammogram, they used a magic marker to mark up my breast. I looked like a medical puzzle. It wasn't until they led me into the room in which they were going to do the actual biopsy that I began to worry.

It was a larger room, set in the basement of the building. In the middle of the room was a gurney with a black rubber mattress. The strange thing about this gurney was that it had a hole in it.

"Let me explain," the doctor said, "You will lie on your stomach, on the gurney with your affected breast in the hole. Once we start, you will not be able to move at all. You won't feel a thing because I will administer a local. We will have to take a lot of pictures."

I wasn't too concerned about the pictures. I was concerned about the table. How in the world were they going to reach the area they needed to access? I guess my look said it all, because the nurse with the sense of humor laughed and answered my unspoken question.

"The table is on a lift. The table will be raised up toward the ceiling and we will be operating beneath you," explained the nurse.

"Oh...," was all I could manage in response.

I was obedient, lying on the table covered with sheets and with my 'affected part' hanging out of the hole. Up, up, up I went, until my rump was just a foot from the ceiling. It is strange for a short person to see a room from the prospective of a common housefly. Up in the air, I could see all the dust balls that the housekeeper - obviously short, too - had missed. I could see the bald spots of the lab tech who kept running in and out with samples. I was up there for a long time. It seemed so long that I swear I had delusional visions. The doctor and the nurse started to look and dress like the mechanics who gave my car its oil changes.

The hardest part was that I couldn't move. According to the nurse, I had to get in a comfortable position and stay there. I laid on the gurney, and the doctor operated. I didn't feel any pain. She took x-rays and each time they took an x-ray, the doctor and nurse would assure me that the radiation was too low to hurt me. Then they would almost knock each other down getting behind the large protective screen.

During the long hours, I lay suspended by the ceiling; the doctor placed a marker, and took samples to send to the lab for biopsies. A marker is a small metal chip that marks the site of the biopsy. It is placed in case the lesion is cancerous and surgery is needed. I floated down to earth only once to take another mammogram. The mammogram would make sure the marker was placed in the right area. In the future, the marker would indicate where the questionable area was located.

I was glad to drive out of there. Never before, despite the kindness of the staff, had I experienced such a strange event. I would never look at a car on a lift in a garage in quite the same way.

Whispers

As a writer, I know the importance of every word. A single word can completely change the meaning of a sentence. Even a word as simple as 'yes' or 'no' can change a meaning or a life. A man gets down on bended knee and asks a girl to marry him. If she says 'no', a door closes, if however, she says 'yes' a lifetime of possibilities open. A prosecutor stands and questions a witness, saying, "Did you kill the victim?" If the witness says 'no', he walks out of the courtroom. If he answers 'yes', he leaves in handcuffs to a limited life in prison.

These are just small examples of the power of simple words. One word can cut like a knife, wounding the receiver. Another word can soothe like a balm. Often, the words and the power they hold are neglected, as if words like paper napkins could be used and thrown away. I know better. As a child, I learned to choose the words I spoke very carefully. I was taught that a word once spoken could never be taken back. The words we choose can either bless or curse.

As a writer of religious fiction, I am well aware of the deeper meaning of words. The gospel of John starts, "In the beginning was the Word, and the Word was with God, and the Word was God."[5] The story of creation says that light, substance and all life came into being only when God spoke. So right from the beginning, God teaches us the power of words. Scientists tell us that the qualities that separate man from the lower animals are the ability to use tools, and the ability to speak.

Language is the main difference. I find this no surprise. For in the second chapter of Genesis, it states, "The Lord God formed man out of the clay of the ground and blew into his nostrils the breath of life, and so man became a living being."[6] Life came from a breath of God, and the very words we breathe carry the power of life.

Poets, who agonize over each word in a line of poetry, have always known this. The shorter the poem, the more importance each word takes on. In seven short words, Sandburg tells us the nature of fog, 'The fog comes on little cat feet." Chosen well, words need not be lengthy. Language has its own nature. Some words are shouts, words like 'help', or 'fire.' When we hear the shout words, we are on alert. There is immediate danger. Our hearts pound and our muscles tense for movement. We go into the fight or flight response and seek protection. Shout words are frightening, but whisper words are even more so.

Imagine yourself watching a horror movie. The maniac killer calls the vulnerable victim and shouts threats at her. Now, imagine the killer calls and whispers those same threats. These whispers generate a deeper, colder type of fear. What does this have to do with us? We all carry whisper words. These words are so deep within us that we may not even notice them. We may only know our reaction to those words. A certain situation makes us uncomfortable or we instinctively avoid certain people or places without knowing why. What are whisper words and where do they come from?

We learn whisper words as children, as adults bend in secret conversation and lower their voices. Whispered words that leak from private conversations spill across to children as adults look resigned to hopelessness. As a child, I walked with my sister the five blocks to the corner. Here we would greet our friends as we waited for the school bus. Neighborhood parents held the hands of the younger children and everyone knew everyone else. Occasionally, a mother just seemed to disappear. Whispers of the adults often leaked the word 'cancer'. I didn't know the meaning; I only knew that the mother was never seen again. It was as if there was this place called cancer and once someone went to the land of cancer there was no return. Later the whispers of the adults at the bus stop would spill the words 'wake' and 'funeral' - whisper words of death. Sometimes our friends - the children of the missing mother - would also disappear.

As children, we never asked about the whisper words. Whisper words, never forgotten, hide in your spirit. I grew to be a nurse. I knew all about cancer. I knew that many people, especially now with all the advances, were cancer survivors. Nevertheless, when I heard the whisper word applied to me, the memory of people who never returned rose from my spirit. Despite our sense of maturity, our spirit holds the whisper words in a place of primal fear. Lessons learned in childhood remain in the spirit despite all adult knowledge to the contrary.

Cancer, CANCER! I held the phone as the doctor droned on. She talked about type, and size and surgery. I could only hear the word 'cancer'. It screamed through my mind but couldn't penetrate it. I said all the proper words by rote. My mind was numb; unable to believe the news. I was the eternal optimist, always full of hope and joy. Now if I couldn't accept it, how would I tell others? Who should I tell?

A strange sensation flooded through me. I didn't want to tell anyone. It was as if by saying it aloud, it would be true. Therefore, my mind deducted by a strange convoluted logic, that if I didn't say it out loud, it wouldn't become true. This strange thought only lasted for a few minutes. My husband, Mike was sitting right there. He knew it was the doctor on the phone. I had to tell him the truth. Hanging up the phone, I turned to see the happy, expectant look on his face. He expected the best. When I told him, his guard fell for just a minute as the look of shock flowed quickly across his eyes and a stoic strength settled in. "You're kidding?" was all he could produce.

I tried to mend the wound he had just received with the words of the doctor. The cancer was caught early. They would check during surgery to see if it had spread. Mike grabbed the words and rephrasing them, smiled and whispered them back to me. He found his positive. Now he wanted to convince me that the gift of optimism I had bestowed on him was true and that he could give that gift back. I had to tell my grown children; they lived with me and would have to know the reason for the surgery. I told my son when he returned from his college classes. Pain and fear crossed his eyes, but like his father, he immediately took the role of optimistic comforter. My daughter was more truthful; she cried.

It took some days to let the reality of cancer sink into my mind. Who should I tell? I didn't want to shock my mother. She had suffered a stroke the year before. She had experienced a miraculous recovery, but still seemed frail and affected. The news might actually harm her. And if I didn't tell her, I decided, I couldn't tell anyone in my family. What would happen if someone had a slip of the tongue? Finding out that her daughter had cancer that way would even be more of a shock. No, I decided, I couldn't take that risk. I had to keep the secret from my sister and two brothers.

And if I didn't tell my family, I certainly couldn't tell my husband's family. What would happen if they ran into one another? It would be only natural for someone to ask how I was doing. It would spread through the family quickly and the one source of information that everyone would turn to would be my mother. No, I decided, no one could know. I did go to my priest. He had suffered from a serious illness, and prayed with me. He also gave me some advice that may have saved my life and which I will refer to later. I told some of my close friends at my prayer group. I didn't want anyone else to know. I guess I was afraid of the reaction.

Everything went fine for a few weeks. Then during a morning Mass, I noticed people whispering. I could swear that the people bent over in whispers were looking at me. Was it my imagination? No, I found out during the Mass that someone, a very good friend with the finest intention, had called to have my name announced at Mass for prayer - so much for secrets! That's the way it is with whisper words like 'cancer.' It is impossible to keep the whispers from drifting on the wind.

The most powerful words, however, are the words we whisper to ourselves. They are like tapes that play constantly in our spirit.

Sometimes, we are unaware of the words we speak to ourselves. My spirit was speaking to me, whispering fear every chance it got. Logic has no place in fear. I had my surgery; a lumpectomy. I knew that I was getting the best treatment. Still, the whispers continued to interrupt my sleep, and depress my days. I knew I had to stop them. Like a recording playing in my mind, during any free moment, the words of fear would sigh. A sense of hopelessness was blanketing me in depression. The more I tried to divert myself, the more the whisper words of fear found me at night. As I lay in my bed, without the noise of daily distractions, the words of fear and anxiety would come. Like a tape recorder that droned on and on, the whisper words of sickness and death would pressure my spirit. It was terrible.

I know that the mind can greatly affect the body. I wanted only positive healing words to flow through my mind and spirit to my body. But what words? I really had to think, believing that each word had to be a word of power. Each word of power had to drip into my spirit replacing the words of harm. The words had to be so strong that they had the power to erase the negative words now playing.

Then, it came to me; they had to be words of expectant healing. What was more powerful then gratitude for a healing already accepted as true? Soon I had them, words of gratitude and healing. Each time a moment came, I repeated to both God and myself, "Thank you Lord for healing me." As these healing words of thanks replaced the words of fear, I had new whisper words. Whisper words that, I believe, did lead to my healing.

Each person must find his or her own healing words. No two people have the same spirit or belief system. People have their individual words of fear to replace. I don't know what the words are for you, but if you want to become a cancer survivor, you have to search for your own whisper words of fear and replace them with positive words of hope and courage. To this day, I whisper, at any given moment, the words: "Thank you Lord, for healing me." What are the words you are whispering to your spirit?

Your Best Friend

I believe God creates each individual for a special life with unique gifts to contribute to the world. I firmly believed this in my mind. Did I live as if I believed? No, I definitely didn't live in the reflection of this enlightened knowledge. It was in my mind but not my heart. Instead of finding my gifts and using them to do what I was created to do, I spent all of time placating others and doing good deeds.

Now of course, there is nothing wrong with doing good deeds. God wants us to help others. However, not to the point of losing one's own way and happiness, and as the years when on, that is exactly what I did. I lost my purpose and myself. I became the person that everyone turned to when needing a favor. Why, did they turn to me? It could be because I never said no. No matter how ridiculous the request, I would do it.

I have always been a person who wants to please everyone. I don't know the psychology behind it. I only know that, even as a child, I would be devastated if someone didn't like me, or if I made someone unhappy. I even thought it was my responsibility to make everyone else happy. Where did this idea start? I'm not sure. I guess I feared what would happen if someone didn't like me.

It is really an egocentric thought. Imagine thinking that you were placed on earth to make everyone else happy. Envision spending all of your time trying not to offend anyone else. That is exactly how I wasted a good portion of my life. Not only is it egocentric to think that you can make everyone else happy but it also prevents you from finding your own peace. If you spend all of your time trying to please others, you lose your way.

It started when I was a child. I would go out of my way to help others and I took it to the extreme. If someone didn't have their lunch, I would not only share my lunch with them, I would give them all my lunch and do without. If someone wanted my candy, I would give all of it. I never worried about myself and that is not a good thing. When Jesus said to "love others, as you love yourself," I somehow missed the 'love yourself part'. I stopped being my own best friend. I denied all my own needs. No matter how tired I was or how many hours I was working, I was the one who would pick you up at the airport. It didn't matter if I only had enough money to make it through the week, if you wanted something I would do without to buy it for you.

Everyone knows someone who behaves as I did. The person you call when you need money is never the rich friend; instead it is the person who always puts your needs ahead of his or her own. When you need a ride, they are at your front door. No appointment they may have had is more important then your schedule. When you need a babysitter, it doesn't matter how they feel, just bring the kids over.

I was a walking heart, just ask me and if it were within my power, I would grant your wish. When a girlfriend cried for hours on the phone about her bad marriage, I would listen to her sorrows even though my own family was patiently waiting for dinner. Oh, that is another thing about people-pleasers; their own family becomes an extension of their nature. In my case, my family had to wait while I catered to others. They should understand, after all, someone needed me. I was being kind. At least that is what I thought. Was I really? No, because I was never kind to myself and treated myself as if I deserved nothing. How sick is that?

I don't think that I was even honest with myself. I wasn't charitable because of innate goodness. I lied to myself. I was operating out of fear. I had a terrible fear of rejection. I couldn't stand the thought of not being accepted. I needed the whole world to love me, but I never loved myself. It wasn't until I had spent all of my time running around for others that I realized that no matter how hard you work, you can't please everyone. There are people who are users, and when you are a people-pleaser, they are drawn to you like a magnet. Two opposites attract and you find yourself exhausted. The users will wear you out and never leave you feeling that you did enough. Now imagine a people-pleaser with cancer. It is a death sentence.

One of the first people I went to speak to was my priest and spiritual advisor. He had suffered through serious illness himself, so I knew that he could help me to make one of the most important decisions of my life. I credit him with guiding me onto the path of saving my own life.

The new doctor, who had discovered the cancer, had a friend who was a surgeon at a local hospital. She strongly encouraged me to make an appointment with her for surgery. Another friend called me and suggested I go to a medical center that specialized in cancer. The medical center treated cancer with a team approach. Each patient is assigned a team of nurses and doctors who meet, discuss, and plan your treatment. On your team is a surgeon, an oncologist who plans your chemotherapy, a radiologist, and a nurse who pulls it all together and explains it all to you.

I was attracted to the second option. I liked the idea of the team. I didn't like the idea of carrying my records from surgeon to radiologist and so on. I was drawn to idea of dealing with a center specializing in cancer. But - wasn't it selfish – after all, the local hospital was closer and more convenient? It would be easier for others to visit me. How could I tell the doctor that I had decided not to take her suggestion and use her friend? These were the thoughts I was mulling over when I went to talk to Father P.

When I explained the decision I had to make, he looked at me as if I had three heads and said, "You have the opportunity to go to the medical center and to the best doctors and you have to think about it? Of course, you will go to the cancer center." In his mind, there was no decision to make. It was such a powerful moment. Right at that instant, my whole outlook on life changed. In a flash, I realized

I now had to learn to put my own needs first.

If you are going to survive the cancer that is exactly what you need to do. Do not - I repeat - do not put anyone or anything ahead of healing yourself. You do not have to please any doctor or any clerk at your insurance company. Now that you have cancer, you have to stop worrying about pleasing others. You are on the most important mission of your life. You are on a mission to save your life.

Find a doctor who is the best; one that you can trust, yes, and check his credentials. If you are a people-pleaser, then you have extra work to do. You have to start thinking of yourself as your own best friend. Would you let your best friend settle for less than the best medical care? What if her life depended on your decision? Well, your best friend's life does depend on it. Once you find a treatment center and doctor that you completely trust, then your work has just begun.

Secondly, you need to educate yourself. Learn everything you can about your cancer. I highly recommend *The Breast Cancer Book*, by Dr. Love. Even though I was a nurse, cancer was not my specialty. This book taught me the lingo - the meaning behind the doctor's words. Without this book, I wouldn't know the questions I needed to ask. Use the Internet, but be careful and check your sources. There are many quacks out there, looking to take your money. Again, you are your own best friend. Your best friend is depending on you to save her life.

I did go to the medical center. I prayed for guidance and ended up with the best surgeon. Wouldn't you do that for anyone who asked you, especially a friend? After my consultation with this surgeon, I decided on a lumpectomy according to his recommendation. I did have fear. Fear told me to get a mastectomy, but my prayers told me to listen to the doctor. I think that most women entertain the thought of removing the breast, maybe even both of them. I didn't want to take a chance. I wanted to live. However, research shows that women do just as well with a lumpectomy followed by chemotherapy or radiation. My doctor was planning both for me. I also had the thought that somehow my body would recover faster from the lesser surgery. I could eat to build up my immune system to fight the cancer. My body could concentrate on fighting the cancer instead of doing massive healing of a major surgery.

The doctor was also going to do a sentinel node dissection. He was going to remove lymph nodes under my arm. The breast drains into these nodes and any sign that the cancer has spread would be discovered by an examination of these nodes. After this surgery and the pathology report, I would have a better idea of where I stood. It is important to learn how to read a pathology report.

Waiting is the hardest part. I found that learning how to read the expected pathology report helped to ease my anxiety. The pathology report gives all the information about your cancer. It can take one to two weeks to be completed. If a week passes and you don't hear from your doctor, don't hesitate to give him or her a phone call. The pathology report will help your doctor decide if you have cancer and what stage you are in. There are five stages of breast cancer and the staging is based on the size of the tumor, and the involvement of the lymph nodes. You should ask for a copy of your pathology report and keep it.

The pathology report will not only tell you what your stage of cancer is, but it will tell you if the cancer is aggressive or slow, if it is estrogen receptive or not. The examination of the nodes will let you know if it has spread beyond the breast. You need this knowledge. It will help you to make all the future decisions that you need to make. Remember, you are the final manager of your care. You need all the facts to make a good decision. Yes, you should listen to the experts. That is why you picked your doctors. But you need to know enough to ask the right questions and decide the best treatments. Your doctor is there to guide you to survival. You are the one who needs to survive.

Start by checking the top and making sure that has your name and the date of your biopsy. The first part of the report should state where the specimen was taken from. It should be the affected breast and possibly the lymph node. It should then contain a clinical history, telling how the cancer was discovered and what type of surgery was done to receive the specimen. It should then list a clinical diagnosis, which is the diagnosis the doctors expected before the biopsy was done. The pathology report is a report of the examination of the cells. There are different tests that are done on the cells and so parts of the report may come in at different times. You may end up with a few different pathology reports that contain different information. Keep them together for your records.

The first part is likely to be the gross examination of the cells. This is the size, weight, and general appearance of the cells that the surgeon sent to the lab. Next will be the microscopic examination, which will describe the type of cells that appear under the microscope. Special test and markers will be done on these cells to describe the kind of cancer and the genes that are involved. These tests will also describe how aggressive the cancer may be. This is the part of the report you will have questions about. Look up any words you don't understand. And don't be afraid to ask questions. These results will determine what your treatment should be. Finally, there will be a general interpretation of the study. Remember, you are learning what you need to know in order to decide the course of treatment that is best. You can't do that unless you understand this report fully.

After you and your doctor receive this report, you will probably have a visit with the doctor to discuss your treatment. This is the time to ask questions. Don't make any decisions that you are not comfortable with or that you do not fully understand.

I have seen women go too far the other way. Armed with a little knowledge, they consider themselves experts. They set up an adversarial relationship with the doctor and fight all of his suggestions. I think that it gives them a sense of control in a situation that seems out of their control. It is important to remember that you picked this doctor for a reason. He has had years of education and experience and what he suggests should carry a lot of weight. Don't make the mistake of thinking that a little bit of research makes you an equal in knowledge. But do ask about everything and weigh each decision carefully. Take all your decisions before a Higher Power; even doctors make mistakes. You are the one who will live with the results of the decisions you make at this most important part of your treatment.

In the end, I found myself stepping out of my personal comfort zone. I had to overcome my own fear of inadequacy and learn to trust my instincts. I had to trust my own power to learn and understand. It was as if I had to remove my decision making process from the fear and emotions that threatened to paralyze me. I had to step outside of myself and think of myself as a person who was under my care. I had to learn to care for myself as I would my best friend. Are you thinking of yourself this way? Are you being your own best friend?

Surgery

I met with the surgeon at the medical center. Grey-haired and dressed in a lab coat, he was experienced and competent. He set my mind at ease the minute I met him. I had an immediate 'gut instinct' that I had made the right choice. We talked about my mammogram and biopsy results. The doctor discussed and explained what he felt the tests told him. We reviewed my medical history and talked about the emotions I felt because of the diagnosis of cancer.

He recommended that I have a lumpectomy. He would remove the cancer and the surrounding tissue. First, he wanted to do a sentinel node dissection. He wanted to remove a lymph node under my right arm and have it tested for cancer. A negative node would indicate that the cancer was still confined to the original site. The first place that breast cancer cells spread to is the axillary's nodes. If my node was positive it would mean that further tests would be needed to see how far the cancer had spread. I wanted to know and yet I was afraid to find out. The test results would help us decide what treatments I needed, but also how much the cancer had spread.

The thought of the cancer spreading really bothered me. I didn't want it in me. I imagined it like an alien invader stalking through my system. In my nightmares, I pictured it growing and expanding. Every little ache and pain now became cancer. When my arthritis hurt, my mind said it was cancer spreading to the bone. When I developed a cough, my imagination just knew the cancer had spread to my lungs. I was full of fear. It felt as if my body was now my enemy and the idea of cancer cells floating around inside me and attaching themselves to different parts really bothered me. I wanted the cancer cut out immediately. I didn't want to wait. The terror I felt told me that the cancer was spreading throughout my body choking the life out of me. The only thing that gave me peace was my faith. It took all the patience I had to wait. I had no choice. I listened to the surgeon and had the node surgery first.

I arrived at five in the morning as instructed. No coffee ran through my veins, yet I was more awake than I had ever been. The heavy-set nurse took me back to the same day surgical area where I was given a hanger with a clothing bag attached and taken to a dressing room. Everything had to go - shoes, socks, the works - into the bag. Hanging up my clothes, I donned the worn-out Johnny coat and strange paper slippers I had been handed. The large paper cap, which looked like a poor shower cap, covered my head.

Dressed in this designer outfit, I headed out to the nurse. Slipping along the floor in my paper shoes, as I tried to hold my Johnny coat closed, I was directed to my room. Each patient awaiting surgery was given a number of a 'room'. The room was just a curtained area with a number attached. Beyond the curtains was a large lounge chair with wheels. The chair was covered in sheets. Settling in, I waited for the nurse to bring my husband. I watched as other patients were prepared for their surgeries.

Soon enough it was my turn. First, they attempted to start an intravenous. They couldn't find a vein. The nurse tried, then her friend. Finally, the anesthesiologist found a vein on in my hand and started the IV. It gave him the chance to explain the type of anesthesia. Apparently, I was going to be awake during the surgery. However, a local would be given so I wouldn't feel any pain. I would also be given a drug so I wouldn't care or worry about what was going on. I was set and ready to go; at least that is what I thought.

The surgeon was the first to notice the rings on my finger. My wedding ring and engagement ring had been on my ring finger for 30 years. As I gained weight over the years of childbirth and home-cooked meals, the rings had just become a part of my hand. I never took them off. The few times I had taken them off for a good cleaning had been a chore. I had to use liquid soap and take my time, swirling and twirling the tight rings slowly up my ring finger until the too small rings would finally come off.

The surgeon was insistent that the rings had to be removed. Apparently, I was to be placed on electric pads that would help monitor my vital signs. There was a danger that an electric shock could occur and any area with metal on it would receive a burn. The rings had to come off and there was no time for me to twirl and whirl them off. The operating room was waiting, so they sent for the 'tool.' Up from the depths of the hospital, a man appeared. He brought the special tool that everyone was patiently waiting for. The tool cut off both my wedding band and my engagement ring. Both rings were given to my husband for safekeeping. With a ring finger naked for the first time in 30 years, I was placed on a gurney and taken to my first surgery.

The anesthesia produced a twilight sleep that left me asleep but vaguely aware of the movement of the surgical team. I was able to answer any questions that the doctor asked me. I could also tell him if I felt any pain and he would administer more medication. Between the doctor's questions and the occasional twinge of pain that awakened me, I dreamt.

In my dreams, I designed a ring to replace my now ruined wedding and engagement bands. Colorful stones and shining bands of gold flowed through my imagination. Finally satisfied, I admired the ring of my thoughts. The dream continued until the surgery was finally over and I heard the nurse calling my name. It felt as if I had been there for hours, but it was really a short surgery. Soon enough I was awake, bandaged and brought back to the recovery room, minus my lymph node and my treasured rings. Within a few days, I would receive the blessed news that the node was negative for cancer. The cancer had not spread and my chance to live became even greater.

My husband waited for me. He would do a lot of waiting over the next year. The nurse who helped me prepare for home, joked, "Now's your chance. No rings, no marriage, now's the time to leave him if you want!" Looking to my husband who had already managed to lose the small wedding band of gold, I smiled. We had many differences, especially at the beginning of our 30 years of marriage. However, like the ring and my finger, we had melded together over the many years. It was too tight a fit. We couldn't be separated.

Eventually, the diamond from my engagement ring would be reset in the ring I dreamed of during my surgery. The diamond was set in the heart of a claddagh ring. A claddagh is an Irish symbol displaying a heart topped with a crown held on the side by two hands. It represents love, friendship and loyalty. I had the diamond set in the heart and the birthstones of both of my grown children in the hands that held the heart. It wasn't expensive, but it was worth everything to me, because it's a ring representing the best part of my life - a loving marriage and two wonderful children. It was a ring of victory, victory in a fight for life against cancer and death. My husband was at my side throughout the year's treatments. He sat beside me through five surgeries, chemotherapy, and radiation. He spent every free moment with me during my hospital stays. Some things are more precious than gold and diamonds.

The Wig

I had three surgeries. Once the lymph node was found to be negative, I had my lumpectomy and had surgery to place a 'port' by the clavicle bone to receive the chemo. I thought that I was prepared. I had been given a lot of material to read about chemotherapy and how best to understand and handle it. One of the suggestions made in a pamphlet I was given, is that you go a purchase a wig - if you plan to wear one - before you start to lose your hair. The reason for this was that it would be easier to match your hairstyle and color if the wig shop could see how you looked before you went bald.

I had never worn a wig. Once I worked the night shift with a nurse who wore a wig every night. There was nothing wrong with her own head of gray hair. She just couldn't be bothered with doing her hair every night and she found it easier to plop a wig on her head. She was in her late sixties but somehow decided that a blonde wig worthy of Madonna would make her look younger. She would apply the shoulder length wig to her head, then pin a large starched nurse's cap to the wig.

Most nurses no longer wear caps because of the inconvenience they cause while giving care. However, this nurse insisted that the wearing the cap gave her the respect of the patients. The weight of the cap would have the wig sliding around her head all night. She would come to work with the wig leaning to the right. As she moved around giving her medication, it would flip to the left. Poring over her charts would cause the cap and the wig to slide forward covering most of her forehead. I spent most of my night waiting for both the wig and the cap to fall off. When she opened the bed curtains, her large cap would tangle in the patient's curtain, further spinning the location of the wig on her head. The sight of this wrinkled nurse with the long blonde curls and spinning cap probably scared or cured many a patient.

I decided from this experience, that I needed help in picking out my wig. Naturally, I called my best friend. We would make buying my wig a day trip that would include lunch. I turned to the phone book as my primary source of wig information. I called and checked prices. Now the prices of wigs can vary as much as the prices of cars. They can start around 100 dollars, and can cost as much as a few thousand dollars. I quickly eliminated the pricier shops. It was, after all, a temporary wig. Armed with the addresses and directions to the varied wig shops, I was ready and on my way to looking good.

We went to the large mall in our area. The wig shop there turned out to be for teenyboppers who wanted wig extensions for the weekend. They were happy to usher out two chubby middle-aged women, before we hurt their image. We started to the next shop on our list. The name of the shop has been changed to protect the innocent, but it was similar to 'Wigs for the Road'. The name was a good indication of what was coming. It turned out to be an old-fashioned shop whose walls were lined with shelves that contained endless cartons the size of shoeboxes. These boxes, and there were thousands of them, held wigs.

The woman took me to the back room and sat me in a spinning beauty parlor chair before a large mirror. She seemed to know her business. The top shelf lining the room contained foam head forms with various wigs. I immediately spotted what I thought was the perfect wig for me. It was brown, like my own hair, of medium length and seemed just right. The sales clerk measured my head and disappeared into the large, mysterious back room that contained thousands of wigs in an impressive inventory. Within minutes, she was back with the wig.

That is when I found out that what looks good on a foam head form doesn't necessarily look good on a real head. The wig I had picked made me look like a time traveler from the fifties. After we stopped laughing, I took a real risk and tried on a blonde, curly wig. This time I looked like Harpo from the Marx brothers. Wig after wig reduced us to tears. It was looking hopeless. My friend started pointing to the turbans and the turban option was starting to take on a more serious meaning. Then suddenly the owner of the wig shop appeared. She had come to see what was causing all the laughter.

Introducing herself, she told me that she was a breast cancer survivor. She had opened the shop to help people like herself. She was now on her fifth round of chemotherapy for her cancer and had not seen her hair for a very long time. She said that when she first got cancer, she couldn't find a decent wig and that is what caused her to open up the business. She went to the back room and appeared again with a wig box. When she pulled the wig out of the box, I was not impressed. The wig was short and feathered. It was a golden brown color and I didn't think it would look good on me. However, when she placed on my head it was the perfect wig. It looked real, even better than my own hair.

"What did the doctor tell you about losing your hair?" she asked.

I smiled and answered, "Oh, she said that I wouldn't lose my hair until the second or third treatment."

"Better buy the wig," she responded, "You'll lose your hair on the seventeenth day."

I left the shop with a foam head form, the wig, and two turbans, sure, that I wouldn't need them for a long while.

Seventeen nights after my first chemotherapy treatment, I was turning over in the middle of the night. I reached up to brush some hair out of my face and woke up in shock. The hair I had brushed out of my face was now in my hand and not at all attached to my scalp. Reaching up in the dark, I took a large clump of hair at the top of my head in my hand and gave it a gentle tug. It easily came loose from my scalp. Even though I was expecting this, it was a big shock.

I sat up stunned. Turning on the light, I checked my pillow. No, there were no loose hairs on it. My scalp had a tingling, sore feeling. I reached up and touched my hair and came away with another bunch of loose hair. It was three o'clock in the morning and as my husband snored peacefully beside me, the thought of going back to sleep and waking up in a bed full of hair suddenly disgusted me.

I plodded barefoot into the bathroom. Looking in the mirror, I simply grabbed the scissors and started cutting off my hair in large clumps and throwing those clumps neatly in the trashcan. When most of the hair I could hold in my hand was chopped off, I went to the closet, grabbed a large garbage bag, my husband's electric shaver, shaving cream and my son's Gillette razor. Going back to the bathroom, I stood on the garbage bag and gave myself a buzz cut. Taking the shaving cream I then gave my head a clean shave, like Mr. Clean.

Looking in the mirror was a shock. It was by now four in the morning and I suddenly realized the extreme measure I had taken without much thought. There is nothing stranger for a woman than to see herself completely bald with a shining scalp. Did I feel depressed about it? No, somehow I was elated about taking control of the situation. I wasn't going to allow chemo or cancer to rob me of hair. I took it off myself. It gave me a great sense of being in command. So much of the cancer experience is beyond your control. Shaving my own head made me feel powerful.

Now I had to see how I good I could make this little chubby woman with no hair look. At four in the morning, I stood in my bathroom applying make-up, loop earrings and a turban. I decided it wasn't so bad. I could start giving crystal ball readings in the morning and get away with it. The turban gave just the right effect. Satisfied with my new look, I returned to my hairless sheets and gave my new wig an introductory nod on my way back to bed. It had been sitting on my dresser, propped on the foam headstand, for the last few weeks. I returned to bed content and fell easily to sleep. After all, my husband would awake to the bigger shock.

Chemotherapy

There is something about the word 'chemotherapy.' It conjures up all kinds of images. For me, the impression was that of a weak, hairless woman who was unable to participate in life. I had visions of a woman who was continuously nauseous and unable to eat. I pictured a person who, while trying to cling to life, was wasting away from the treatment. This image was pulled up from the memory of the many 'chick' flicks of brave women who found new homes for their children while they slowly died of cancer. One of my best movie memories was of a made-for-TV flick in which a young woman who was dying of cancer actually spent her last days finding a new wife for her clearly inept husband.

I looked across the table at my husband devouring his dinner and realized that the most important quality he seemed to need in a wife was someone who could cook enough to satisfy a voracious appetite. No woman with tendency to cook healthy food would do. He was a meat-and-potatoes type of guy. He liked to eat, as we say in Jersey, diner style with the meat and potatoes on the main platter and the useless vegetables on the side. I thought of my friends who also liked to eat and realized that most of them had impatient tendencies that would lead them to murder or divorce my husband within a year. When God made two people to go together, it was hard to make another fit. I decided that I had better survive the chemo. Who else would know how to cook for him?

It wasn't that I didn't care about my husband's health. Many years ago, his doctor called and was very concerned that I start cooking healthy. My husband's cholesterol was off the chart. I ran out to the local bookstore and purchased every book on low-fat cooking. I ran to the supermarket to buy all the right ingredients for the low-fat meals in the books. For weeks, I presented him with the strange new foods, and he smiled and ate whatever I put in front of him. It wasn't until I went out to his pick-up truck, looking for something that I found out why he was so satisfied with the skimpy meals. His front seat and the floor of his truck were littered with fast food wrappers from the greasiest joints that lined the highways of his ride home. He had been arriving at my meals with a full belly.

I appreciated that I had to take another approach. I started to cook his favorite meals again. I thought it was better to have him eat home-cooked meals instead of the poor quality fast foods he had been sneaking. I did a little research. I substituted some of my former ingredients with skim milk and low-fat cheese. I started grinding flax seeds and slipping them into his meatloaf and burgers. He never noticed the difference and his cholesterol returned to normal without the need of medication. Sometimes a little change is better than a lot.

That is not what I expected from chemotherapy. I thought it would completely change my life. I had the media's image of the drug therapy and I hoped that I was about to be proven wrong. When I met my oncologist, she was a tiny, upbeat soul with a loving smile. She explained everything carefully to me. She told me of the research she was doing in her field and asked me if I would be interested in participating in the study. After a few moments of thought and prayer, I decided that I would. If I had to 'suffer' through this treatment, I reasoned that I might as well do some good for others. It made me feel as if I were a bigger participant in my care. It gave me a sense of control.

The treatment was to consist of three drugs - 5-Fluorouracil, Cyclophosphamide, and Epirubicin - given intravenously in six sessions. The chemotherapy was scheduled to be given in three-week intervals. The drugs were very caustic and could damage the skin if, when given by a regular IV, the line infiltrated (pulled out of the vein} and the medication leaked into the soft tissue. Since I had veins that were hard to reach, when I was given the option, I decided that I wanted a central line or 'port' to receive the medication. A port is a small, round disc made of plastic or metal. It is surgically implanted under your skin. A catheter connects the port to a large vein. My port was surgically placed under the skin on the right side of my chest right by my clavicle bone. It never hurt, in fact most of the time the skin around the port felt numb. It was about two inches across and made the experience of receiving chemotherapy much easier than it might have been without it.

The nurse at the medical center would insert a needle into the port to give me chemotherapy or draw blood. This needle was left in place for chemotherapy treatments and meant that I didn't need to have the nurse searching for a vein that may have or may not have sustained the treatments. Agreeing to the port was one of the best decisions that I made during my treatment. The main danger of the port was infection of the site, and the site had to be kept clean at all times. However, once the surgical site healed, I was able to shower and go about my business with moderate care of the site.

The first day of my scheduled treatment, I arrived with my husband and my port at the medical center. I was led to a large room that contained numerous 'rooms' with Geri-chairs much like the surgical waiting area. I was very anxious, not knowing what to expect from the toxic chemicals that I was about to receive. The nurse drew blood from the port and it was sent for testing. The tests had to be back before the chemotherapy was given. The treatment itself was easy but I found myself dizzy and slightly nauseous afterward and was happy that my husband could drive me home. There were so many women there alone. It occurred to me that driving and staying with a patient who is receiving chemotherapy would be a great service ministry. I couldn't imagine how alone a woman could feel as she was given these strong drugs and left to get home alone.

One of the ways that I controlled my fear of the chemo

drugs was to think of them as antibiotics. I thought of the cancer as an infection that had invaded my body. The chemotherapy was the 'antibiotic' to get rid of the infection. It may seem silly but antibiotics are such a normal thing. We take them without question, because, while we know that they have side effects, we expect them to get rid of the infection. We consider the side effects to be well worth the trouble and know that we will recover with the temporary inconvenience. There is no fear involved in taking antibiotics.

While it may seem silly to think of chemo drugs this way, it helped me immensely. It took away the fear as I watched the caustic drugs dripping into my body. Thinking of these potentially harmful drugs as run-of-the-mill antibiotics helped me to see the drugs as something healing rather then as something to fear. The silly game I played with my mind actually took the fear away.

The hospital did give medication to control the aftereffects and I faithfully took it. Apart from the slight nausea and the dizzy feeling, I was doing well. Since the side effects were not happening, I continued my life - minus my hair, of course - as if I weren't receiving chemo. I continued my chores on the farm, such as feeding and caring for the animals, handling bales of hay, and collecting the eggs as if nothing new was happening to me. Even though it would have made medical sense for me to stay away from crowds, I felt so good that I ignored the fact that my immune system was compromised. I decided that I could go to Mass. I was so thankful that the cancer had been caught early, against all odds. I was even grateful to be going through the chemo in the winter. I couldn't imagine wearing a wig in the summertime. I felt really good and didn't see any point in acting like a chemo patient.

I worked on the farm and went to crowded Masses at church without fear. I did tell the people at church that I couldn't shake their hand during the 'peace be with you' part of the Mass, but that was the least of the problems in my parish. We do as the Bible says; greet each other with hugs and kisses. In spite of my caution, the hugs and the kisses increased as everyone who now knew I had cancer wanted to give me their love and pray 'hands-on' over me. Out of everyone, only one person, my friend Bonnie, remembered my germ concern. I was again grateful that it was winter, as I could keep my gloves on during the Mass.

My first warning that things were going wrong was the day of the Super Bowl. I had my daughter's fiancé over to watch the game. I decided that there was no reason for me to change my habits. Of course I would cook. I decided that hot Reuben sandwiches would be easy to make. As I stood at the stove, heating up the sauerkraut and corned beef, my knees started to wobble. I felt myself breaking out in a cold sweat. As the cheers from the family room grew in volume, the kitchen started to spin.

I turned everything off and headed for the bathroom. I made it to the bathroom off the master bedroom. I didn't want anyone to know that I was ill. I spent the next 45 minutes trying not to pass out cold in the bathroom as the nausea and dizziness overtook me. This was not a good thing. It passed, and I went out and served the Reuben sandwiches as if nothing had happened. There were some inquiries, but I brushed them off. I was retreating into my former behavior of thinking I could take care of myself. It was a sign of things to come.

Night Visitors

Chemotherapy and radiology both affect the immune system of the body. In other words, they compromise the exact system your body needs to fight and destroy the cancer cells. The immune system is naturally equiped to destroy the cancer cells that are invading your body, so it is not an easy decision to take drugs that will destroy the natural system to heal the body. The immune system protects the body against infections by bacteria and viruses. In many ways, the immune system is especially important to cancer patients.

Both chemotherapy and radiation cause a drop in the number of white cells made in the bone marrow. Some of the cells of the immune system can recognize cancer cells and kill them but not enough to end the threat of the cancer. This effect means that it is difficult to defeat cancer with just your own immune system.

The problem with using the drugs to kill the cancer is that it leaves your body open to numerous infections. A cancer patient needs to be careful; it is difficult to fear the very family and friends you need to keep your spirit high. However, many infections can be caused by germs that normally live on the patient's skin and those 'good' bacteria that normally reside in your body. Usually these germs are harmless, often even protective by fighting off more harmful bacteria. However, now that you are being treated, your defenses have been weakened and you will be, for a while 'off-balance.' It happens that the normal flora in your body can now attack and cause a severe infection.

The white blood cells in your body perform many functions

to defeat the bacteria, virus, and fungi that attack your health. "Chemotherapy drugs target cancer cells, but they can affect healthy cells as well, including infection-fighting white blood cells," states Nicole M. Kuderer, M.D., a hematology-oncology fellow at Duke and lead author of the publication, Duke Health. "When patients' white blood cell counts drop too low, they are at risk for dangerous infections that can cause death."[7] At the first sign of an invasion, the white blood cells rush to the site of the infection. They grab hold of the invading property and swallow up the invaders, sort of like Pac-Man for those old enough to remember him. The white cells kill the bacteria they have swallowed by producing various chemicals. Three thousand to six thousand per militre of blood is the normal count of white blood cells.

When I received my first treatment, I felt weak and dizzy but the feeling soon passed. I felt better than I had expected to. I guess it gave me a sense of confidence. I took the medications to control the aftereffects of the chemo and seemed to do okay. I rested a little, but I felt so good that I ignored any signs of infection and went about my business. I didn't realize that a lower white blood cell count not only causes infections, but it also makes the infection move rapidly through your body. If you get a fever or other sign of infection you should go immediately to your physician and get some antibiotics. The antibiotics could save your life. That is exactly what I didn't do.

I continued to live my life as if I didn't have cancer. I ignored the fact that I was on chemo. I exposed myself to many germs that I could have avoided. The most pronounced effect of the drugs I was receiving was a sense of being detached. It felt as if I were standing outside of myself and watching myself live my life. It is a difficult side effect to explain. I didn't feel depressed or worried, I just felt so detached. This feeling increased when I took the medication to control the side effects of the chemotherpy. I attributed the feeling to those drugs.

I managed with the help of my oncologist to avoid the nausea and vomiting that is so often attributed to these heavy cancer-fighting drugs. However, as I finished my third course of chemo, things went radically wrong.

It was a Wednesday when I first felt as if I was a little short of breath. I took it easy and decided that I just needed a rest. By Friday, I was really suffering with the shortness of breath. I felt as if I couldn't get enough air in. I didn't want to be a 'complainer' or a baby. I decided that I would tell the nurse about it at my chemo treatment next week. It was a Saturday, when I tried to walk the six feet from my bathroom to my bedroom door and couldn't make it. I had to sit down on the side of my bed and try not to pass out from the lack of oxygen. Realizing that I was in real trouble, I had my husband call the oncologist. She told me to get to the nearest hospital immediately. I listened to her, but for other reasons wished I had taken the longer drive to the cancer institute. I was in full-blown pneumonia.

I was put on oxygen and monitors immediately. My husband stayed with me as I spent the night in the emergency room. I was transferred to the floor in the morning. Little did I know that the next 10 days would be the hardest days I spent with the cancer.

I didn't have access to my regular oncologist, or surgeon. I was assigned doctors I didn't know. That turned out to be both a blessing and a curse.

I guess I looked even worse than I felt. I was pale and weak and unable to walk to the bathroom without losing my breath. I was assigned an internist. He was the blessing. He was the type of physician who wanted not only to cure me, but he also wanted to know what had caused the pneumonia. His curiosity and caring was so refreshing that he has been my doctor ever since. I love someone who has a passion for his work.

What I didn't know was that I would be at the mercy of so many who didn't know what they were doing. I looked bad. I don't think I realized how close I was to death. By now, my mother knew about my illness. I told her when the surgery was over. I knew I couldn't hide the loss of my hair from her. My sister and mother came to visit me in the hospital. I didn't know that when they left, they felt they might not see me alive again. I looked that bad.

The doctors who were assigned my case were, for the most part, kind and caring. However, most of them decided that the cancer had spread. They were convinced that I had developed lung cancer. I was sent for MRI's and x-rays.

I continued to have trouble breathing, even though I was given inhalation therapy twice a day and sustained on oxygen. Late one evening as I was dozing in my bed, I awoke with the feeling that someone was watching me. There at the bottom of my bed was a short doctor, one that I had never seen before. He was dressed in green scrubs and looked up from the chart he was holding, to me. I sat in my bed with my turban on, wondering who this doctor was. He didn't introduce himself. Instead, he started with an accusation, "Do you smoke?"

"I used to, I quit 11 years ago." I answered.

"You probably have lung cancer. We can't see it with the tests. We'll have to 'crack you open' to find it."

I remained silent, but my mind answered, *You and what army?* I knew I wasn't about to let this doctor touch me. I was a nurse. I didn't have any fear over what this doctor said. I knew he would never operate on me. He closed the chart and left. I don't know if he was waiting for a hysterical reaction. Too bad for him, he had just met someone who knew he was an idiot. Nevertheless, it got me to thinking. How did a person who didn't have a medical background deal with the many people who, without much thought, said the most horrible things?

As I was going through my illness, I had people say, "Who knew huh, who knew you would die this way?" Others would say things like, "Oh my aunt died of breast cancer just last year. Yeah, the doctors told her she would make it, just like you."

Most of the people who make these stupid statements mean well. Many people get nervous around sick people. They don't know what to say. They ramble and in that nervous ramble, they make the idiotic statements. Have mercy on them, they are really trying to comfort. They are just failing badly.

There are others, however, just like this doctor who mean to hurt you. It almost seems that they like to kick you when you are down. They want to make sure that you know that getting cancer is somehow your fault. I can't help but think that it is their own fear that drives them. Somehow, if they can convince themselves that you got cancer because of something you did, they feel they don't have to fear getting cancer themselves. That is not true, of course. Cancer happens to those who do everything to prevent it. No one is exempt. Imagine the fear that would drive a person to talk and think in such a way. After you make sure that none of these thoughtless statements have taken away your peace, pray for the person. After all, it is much better to have cancer and be at peace, then to be healthy and full of fear.

My worst experience was the lung biopsy that the doctors ordered to see if the cancer had spread. I had to be awake for it. My throat was numbed, but still my gag reflex was triggered as the tube was passed down through my trachea and into my lung. I lay there, feeling the instrument moving around in my lung. I felt so trapped and I closed my eyes to pray that it would end. It was truly the worst experience I suffered in all of my cancer treatment. The Lord was good, however, and the lung biopsies came back negative. I didn't have lung cancer; just a severe case of pneumonia.

I had many visitors while I was in the hospital. One of my favorite visitors was Father P. First, I received a phone call. Father P was in the lobby of a different hospital, 30 miles away. I gave him the bad news. Someone had given him the wrong information. I felt terrible that I missed his visit. To my surprise, he arrived at my hospital bed within 45 minutes. He prayed over me and anointed me with oil. He never said it but I think he performed the Sacrament of the Sick. It used to be called Last Rites.

It simply never occurred to me that I might die. The night the strange doctor came, I almost faltered in my belief that I would defeat this cancer. I pulled out my Bible and read the 23rd Psalm at least five times. I knew that God was with me. I didn't believe it was His Will that I should die.

I did have a decision to make. I had to decide, after this terrible infection, if I wanted to continue with the chemotherapy. This was not an easy decision to make. My cancer had been caught in an early stage. It had not spread beyond the breast. However, it was high-grade cancer, which means it was an aggressive form of cancer. I didn't tell anyone what I was thinking. I prayed about it. Every time I thought of getting another course of chemo I would actually get nauseous. I took this as a sign and decided to end the chemo. This was a purely personal decision. I canceled the next three courses of chemo that I had scheduled. Was this a 'right' decision? Only time would tell. I was sure it was right for me. I was to start the radiation treatments as soon as the pneumonia was gone.

At some point, the intravenous antibiotics started to work and the pneumonia was going away. I was weaned off the oxygen and allowed home on the tenth day. When I got home, the first thing I noticed was that my children had taken a large stuffed Pink panther animal and sat it in 'my' chair in the family room. They had dressed the stuffed animal in my nightgown, slippers, and wig. She - an imitation me - was sitting next to my husband watching TV. After I stopped laughing, they explained that my husband would look at my empty chair and feel so lonely. They just had to give him a companion. It's sad that I could be replaced by such a passive creature. The only one who knew it wasn't really me seemed to be my Labrador retriever, Gracie. She did nothing but growl at the phony who tried to take my place.

Of Fat and Fiber

I realized - after I received the news of having cancer - my body was just a disease waiting to happen. I was overweight. Okay, I was fat. I had all the expectations of getting heart disease or diabetes. What I never realized was that fat is one of the major factors in developing breast cancer, especially after menopause. This was not something I knew, nor do I think most women know of the connection.

I think most women, like myself, always picture cancer victims as bald and emaciated. The media promotes the thin image of cancer victims wasting away. While that may be true for the final stages of a terminal patient, it is not an accurate picture of the vast majority of women at risk of having the most common form of breast cancer.

The most prevalent kind of breast tumor is an estrogen-receptive tumor. It is fed by the estrogen present in the woman's body. Eighty-percent of the breast cancer diagnosed in this country is estrogen receptive. That is why, in treatment, most women are given a regimen of anti-estrogen drugs that work at reducing the level of estrogen in the body.

Estrogen is a valuable hormone that does great work in the body. It drives growth and development during puberty and causes the secondary growth of the uterus and breast. It protects women from heart disease by promoting 'good' cholesterol instead of 'bad' cholesterol. It softens the bloods vessels and keeps them from stiffening with age. This helps prevent blood clots.

Estrogen also protects a woman's bone by promoting the absorption of calcium from the bloodstream. By doing so, it helps prevent the bone loss that can lead to arthritis and fracture. New studies have linked estrogen with increased mental alertness. There is some evidence that estrogen promotes the creation of new connections between the brain cells. These cells are thought to be responsible for memory and thoughts.

Estrogen, like cholesterol, can be divided into different components. What is important to understand is that there is good estrogen and bad estrogen. The body has estrogen receptors throughout the systems. The breast is a major estrogen receptor. An estrogen receptor is like a lock in a door that only a certain key will fit; in this case the hormone estrogen. The important thing is to have enough of the good estrogen in the bloodstream to fit most of the locks and have most of the bad estrogen eliminated by the body.

Estrogen remains in the bloodstream for a day after being produced. It circulates around the bloodstream looking for a receptor to link on to. If it doesn't find a receptor it moves from the bloodstream into the liver and then from the liver to the bowel to be eliminated. It is easy to understand that having good estrogen keys to fill all of the locks will prevent the bad estrogen from being accepted by those locks. It is also easy to see that eliminating the bad estrogen as quickly as possible is the best way to prevent cancer or a recurrence of a tumor.

Before we talk about what causes good and bad estrogen, we need to understand how having too much estrogen causes breast cancer. Studies of the levels of estrogen in a woman's blood give us a direct link to the development of breast cancer. The higher the level of estrogen, the higher the risk of breast cancer and yes, it is that simple. It is such a strong link that the development of anti-estrogen drugs given to women as part of their recovery has greatly increased their chances of becoming cancer survivors instead of cancer victims. However, this is only part of the picture.

We need to understand how estrogen is produced in the body. The ovaries and the adrenal glands produce estrogen. I never realized or knew is that estrogen is also both produced and stored by fat cells.

In fact, the higher the number and size of the fat cells in the body, the higher the level of estrogen floating around in the bloodstream looking to key into the receptor locks.

At first, I was devastated to realize that the most important thing I needed to do was to reach a normal weight. However, I was also excited to know that I could do something to prevent the cancer from coming back and that thing was to lose the weight. Suddenly I had some sense of control. I was given something to do that was within my grasp. Getting back to the normal weight for my height might actually save my life by eliminating the fat cells that were producing the estrogen my cancer craved.

Lowering the level of estrogen in my bloodstream was possible because I could lose weight and take the anti-estrogen drug that my physician recommended I take for five years. Studies showed that after five years the drugs has little effect in reducing the recurrence of breast cancer. To my way of thinking that meant, I needed to reach a normal weight as soon as possible but definitely within the years I was taking the anti-estrogen drug. It gave me an incentive and a window. I wanted to live.

There are also chemical estrogens that are similar in molecular structure to natural estrogen. These strong chemical estrogens are so similar to natural estrogen that they can lock into the estrogen receptors in the breast. The danger is that the receptors in the breast magnify the power of these estrogens increasing their effect greatly. These chemical estrogens are the pesticides in our food and water supplies. They are extremely toxic and pesticides found in food, water, and even those for outside use should be avoided completely.

But there is more than lowering the level of estrogen in the bloodstream that I needed to do. Estrogen is like cholesterol. There is a good or 'weak' estrogen and a bad or 'strong' estrogen. It was important to me to lower the amount of strong estrogens by replacing them with weak estrogens. The easiest way to do this was with food. To understand what food has to do with it, it is necessary to understand how strong and weak estrogens are introduced to the body.

Strong or bad estrogens trigger a 'spark' of power when they enter the lock of the breast receptor. That spark tells the cell to multiply and increase. If the spark is strong, the change is more pronounced. If the spark is weak, the message to increase and multiply is much weaker. Now imagine the strong estrogen locking into a single cancer cell and damaging the DNA. It can create or increase a tumor. The best prevention is to avoid filling your bloodstream with strong or bad estrogen. This is directly linked to the kind of fat you take in.

A recent 15 year study done by the Harvard School of Medicine followed 90,000 nurses. It was discovered that those who ate red meat five times a week had a 42 percent increase in the chance of developing estrogen receptive cancer over those whose intake was decreased.[8] Today, meats are loaded with hormones and antibiotics. Many of the farmers actually inject estrogen into their cows and chickens to increase their fat production and weight. This raises their income as these animals are sold by weight, while harming the consumer. Even the animals that don't receive the injections of hormone are fed grain that is supplemented with the hormone or other estrogen producing ingredients. Knowing this and the price of organic meats, made giving up eating meat the best choice for me. I am lucky because I live on a small farm. I have free-range chickens that I feed only organic grain. I can easily get some of my protein from the eggs my chickens produce.

However, even if you are able to afford organic meats, it is better to reduce or completely eliminate meat from your diet. Meat and organic proteins contain a large amount of Omega-6 fats, which trigger the fat cells of your own body to produce estrogen. I felt it was best not to take any chances. It is not only possible to get sufficient protein from beans, nuts, soy, and organic dairy products, but these nutrition-filled foods also eliminated many Omega-6 fats from my diet as well. The replacements increase the fiber in my diet that also removes the estrogen that my body produces.

You would think that once the estrogen is eliminated from your liver into your bowel it would be taken care of, but that is not always the case. The hormone can be easily reabsorbed through the bowel wall and back into the bloodstream. This danger can be eliminated by fiber. A large amount of fiber binds the estrogen to itself and keeps it from being reabsorbed. It also quickens the elimination of estrogen. A low-fat vegetarian diet with high fiber is the best way to prevent excess estrogen. The type of fat in your diet is equally important.

The same type of fat that is good for your heart is the same type of fat that helps prevent cancer. Saturated fat, the type that comes from meat and lard increases not only your bad cholesterol but also the strong and bad estrogen. Trans-fatty acids such as margarine and hydrogenated oils also produce the strong or bad estrogens. It is a slam-dunk when it comes to your health. Saturated fats and trans-fatty acids can kill you. However, your body does need fats - good fat such as the oils found in fatty fish as salmon and mackerel. Olive oils should be substituted for butter or margarine. These sources of oil give your body Omega-3 which will both raise your good cholesterol and good estrogen

A diet high in fiber and low in bad fat will help you lose weight and live a longer, healthier life. Many of us know this, but make excuses for our diets. Well, if you have breast cancer, it is time to stop thinking about it and time to start acting. Life is worth it. And when you change your diet you will find out that you really enjoy eating the right way.

Taking the time to feed your body with healthy food makes you feel better. Losing weight gives you even more energy. And here's another bonus. Studies show that those women who exercise regularly have less cancer recurrence than those who are sedentary. See how it all works together. But it's not just about giving up certain foods. It is about adding other important foods to your diet. Adding the food that God created is the key to giving the body what it needs to both fight and avoid cancer.

Vegetables, Fruits, and Nuts

Antioxidants are foods that fight off the free radicals that flow through our bloodstream each day causing damage to our cells. The damage that free radicals cause over time results in oxidation to the nucleus of our cells, damaging the DNA, our information strand that tells the cells what to do.

In the case of cancer, the fractured DNA tells our cells to start proliferating. Usually these cells are defective, and push other healthy cells out of the way to make room for their own growth. Often, they kill the 'normal' cells so that they have room to grow. They form a tumor or a growth that unchecked will take over the body of the person involved. Small groups of cells will break off, traveling through the bloodstream until they find another organ or cavity to attach to and start a new tumor or growth.

How can you stop this disease called cancer? It is difficult and painful. It is better to prevent it from ever happening. Let's get back to the source. How do you stop those free radicals from damaging the cells to begin with? The answer is antioxidants.

Antioxidants are called 'anti' because they prevent the oxidation that causes the very free-floating radicals that damage the DNA and cause cancer. The source of these antioxidants is mainly fruits and vegetables. However, not all fruits and vegetables are alike. Some are so packed with the essential antioxidants that no woman fighting breast cancer can afford to ignore them.

How does someone who has always been on a typically American diet of meat and potatoes change his or her way? I thought at first that I could make a gradual change. I would add a few fruits and vegetables to my diet and reduce the amount of red meat that I ate. This didn't work. I found myself quickly going back to my old habits. I soon realized that if I was going to do this I had to start just eating the right way.

First, I studied all the data out there on diet and cancer. Before I changed my eating habits, I had to convince my mind that I was really doing the right thing. I read books and looked up research on the Internet. I started to look at my food in a different way; I began to think of it as medicine - something I needed to 'take' to fight the cancer cells in my body.

That's when it clicked; it wasn't about giving up food. It was about eating the foods that would help me heal. What I found was that when I ate enough of the food that would fight the cancer, there wasn't any room for the bad food. I knew that I had to make a complete change, not a gradual one. I decided to eat the foods that would fight the cancer and that change has made all the difference to me.

What are these foods? The research is extensive and weighty. I will not go into the research that has been done nor the ongoing studies that continue. That you can do for yourself. I discovered that certain foods had specific qualities to fight cancer. I will list some of the big hitters here for you.

Tomatoes contain lycopene, a rare carotenoid that studies reveal fight all kinds of cancer, including breast cancer. Lycopene also prevents macular degeneration and cataracts. Lycopene is a pigment that gives tomatoes their characteristic red color. It is one of hundreds of carotenoids that color fruits and vegetables red, orange or yellow. Of these pigments, the most familiar is beta-carotene, which is found in carrots.

In the body, these pigments capture electrically charged oxygen molecules that can damage tissue. Because of this they are called antioxidants.

Lycopene has been the focus of much attention since 1995, when a six-year study of nearly 48,000 men by Harvard University found that men who ate at least 10 servings of foods per week containing tomato sauce or tomatoes were 45 percent less likely to develop prostate cancer. The study also found that those who ate four to seven servings per week were 20 percent less likely to develop the cancer. That research was published in the Journal of the National Cancer Institute. Subsequent research has found that lycopene also reduces the amount of oxidized low-density lipoprotein – the so-called bad cholesterol – and therefore may reduce the risk of heart disease.[9]

Tomatoes also contain the antioxidant glutathione, which helps boost the immune system. Using your own immune system to fight cancer is the best way I can think of. Cooked tomatoes release more of the desired antioxidants.

Therefore, tomato paste, sauce, etc. is good to include in your diet. Lycopene is fat-soluble so it is best absorbed if take with a good oil like olive oil.

Garlic is packed with antioxidants. The sulfur in garlic has healing properties. For centuries, men have treasured garlic. Now we know that they had good reason. It fights cancer and heart disease. It lowers cholesterol and free radicals in the blood. It has been known to reduce blood pressure. So far, we have the makings of a really great Italian meal. Just no meatballs and sausage please, substitute whole wheat pasta for semolina. Make a great pasta primavera with a ton of broccoli, carrots and mushrooms in the sauce and you have a truly great cancer fighting meal. However, garlic and tomatoes can be added to almost anything to add flavor. Never skimp on either.

Now why did I add carrots, broccoli, and mushroom to my meal? It is because these too, have powerful antioxidants that fight cancer. Cruciferous vegetables such as broccoli, cauliflower, Brussels sprouts, and cabbage contain a compound called indole-3-carbinal. This powerful antioxidant breaks down estrogen in the body. I make sure that I have a healthy portion of one or two of these vegetables each day. These vegetables reduce the risk of estrogen-produced tumors. These vegetables have other antioxidants that fight cancer.

Carrots, yams, and sweet potatoes contain a lot of beta-carotene which reduce a wide range of cancers. They contain a substance called falcaronol that researchers believe slow the growth of cancer cells. This falcaronol is only found in raw carrots, it is destroyed by cooking. Therefore, have raw carrots in all your salads. I like to use 'carrot chips' (raw carrots cut into chip size) to dip some tomato salsa as a snack. I also used cooked carrots in soups and as a side dish. I often have half a yam or sweet potato sprinkled with cinnamon as a snack. These healthy snacks satisfy my sweet tooth and take the place of all the processed snacks that do harm to my body.

Berries contain so many nutrients it is almost impossible to list them all. Full of fiber, vitamins, antioxidants, and minerals, they provide the body's immune system with a powerful boost. The compounds in berries protect the body from free radicals by actually sweeping the free radicals up before they can damage the cells. I have a full serving of berries each morning to start my day. I vary the type of berry because each berry has different cancer fighting properties. I add blueberries, raspberries, strawberries or blackberries to my steel-cut oatmeal or whole grain cereal in the morning. I eat them mixed with nuts as a snack. I add them to salads. I believe the best way to fight cancer is to make my body so full of antioxidants that it is inhospitable to free radicals and toxins.

I am also sure to add a teaspoon of crushed flax seed to my cereal in the morning. Flax seeds are high in omega-3 fatty acids which is a great replacement for the fat that actually promotes cancer. They also have been shown to lower cholesterol and prevent heart disease. Flax seeds are also full of antioxidants. I buy mine pre-crushed from my health food store. They have to be refrigerated, but I find that I am more likely to use them if I don't have the extra step of grinding the seeds each time.

I am a coffee drinker in the morning who will not give up my beloved cup of coffee. However, in the afternoon and in the evening, I switch to tea. Studies have found that tea - both black and green - contain polyphenols that seem to stop cancer cells from dividing. These polyphenols are also found in red grapes, red wine, and olive oil.

Studies have suggested that tea and its healthy compounds prevent many types of cancer. So experiment with different flavors. I carry my favorite vanilla tea bags around me, so I can have a few cups a day.

I have switched to using olive oil for all my cooking. Some research has suggested that a compound in olive oil called oleic acid is effective in killing the Her2/nea protein, which seems to be a major factor in the growth of breast cancer cells.

Mushrooms, especially, shitake, maitake, and reishi, contain polysaccharides that are powerful compounds. These compounds build up the body's immune system. A strong immune system fights the free radicals that cause cancer. Try adding mushrooms to soup, salads or on top of that vegetable burger you're having for lunch. Mushrooms have been found to have a compound called lectin, which attacks cancer cells and prevents them from multiplying. Mushrooms can actually stimulate the production of interferon in the body. I even like to substitute a large mushroom for meat in a whole-wheat sandwich.

A diet rich in Omega-6 fatty acids can promote the growth of malignant breast cancer tumors. Adding Omega-3 to the diet blocks this effect. Fish oil is an effective way to get the Omega-3 in your body. Women who practice a diet with high fatty fish have a much smaller incident of cancer. It is difficult to get all the fish oil that you need so taking a supplement is something to consider. I take three fish oil capsules a day and order salmon when I go out to eat.

Going out to eat can be a problem. You really don't know how the food is being cooked or prepared. I do the best I can. In my world going out to eat is a given. I eat out for lunch or dinner at least three or four times a week. I have had to learn to accommodate my dietary needs. I order pasta primavera and have no problem asking the waiter if whole-wheat pasta can be substituted. Many restaurants now have whole-wheat pasta and many more will follow if we keep asking. I order salmon and high quality soups or salads. On a rare occasion I get a turkey or chicken burger on a whole-wheat bun. It is not as hard as you think to follow a diet that is healthy for you.

Of course eating food you have prepared yourself is best. So, what diet do I follow? I usually follow a high-quality vegetarian diet. I look at my plate and know I am doing well when I see so many varied and bright colors staring back at me. Green and red vegetables, orange fruit, brown rice with nuts. I try a new fruit or vegetable each week. I create new recipes that replace all the junk food that I used to eat.

Scientists are only beginning to know the benefits of certain vegetables and fruits. I believe that God has placed cancer-fighting compounds in natural and healthy plants that we still know nothing about. Therefore, I eat tons of mushrooms and vegetables. I treat myself to varied fruits and nuts.

I bake my own whole-wheat bread. Did you ever notice that the bread you bake yourself gets hard after only one day? That is because you haven't added the tons of preservatives that store-brought bread has. I find it easy to make because my mother gave me a bread-making machine. I make my bread, cut it up in portions and freeze it until I need it. If this is too hard for you, just buy your bread from a real bakery. They throw their bread out after one day. There is a good reason for that. Bread without preservatives goes stale unless it is frozen.

There are other foods too numerous to mention that will help in your fight against cancer. Even certain spices like rosemary and turmeric have anti-cancer properties. I eat salmon when I go out. I stick to a vegetarian diet at home. You can still eat badly as a vegetarian. Don't make the mistake of giving up meat and loading up on carbohydrates and junk food. I eat many fruits and vegetables with a small amount of whole grains. The research I did led me to take a good multi-vitamin each day. There is mounting evidence that B and D vitamins fight cancer. Along with my Arimidex each day, I take my calcium and fish oil capsules. I make sure I take my calcium separately as this can impair the absorption of the other nutrients and vitamins.

A strange thing happened to me when I started eating this way. I not only gained a sense of control, I started to lose weight. Perhaps this is what was wrong all along. Somewhere along the way, I had stopped eating what was good; the things that God had provided. I had stuffed myself with fatty, sugary, preservative-laden, junk food. It took cancer to make me stop. I continue to lose weight at a healthy clip and I am secure that I am doing my best to stay alive.

When my diet changed, I tried to create tasty new recipes that my family would love. It is hard to cook two different dinners for a family and I knew that cooking two separate meals wouldn't last. I would fall into my old habits unless I could get my husband to eat healthy without realizing he was doing so. I enjoyed creating these recipes and I encourage you to do the same. Experiment with the spices that you like. Make it a game and try to cook the foods that fight cancer in a new and delicious way.

I have included these recipes in the back of the book just to get you started. Once you realize how delicious these nutritious cancer-fighting meals taste, you won't feel deprived at all. You will notice that in some recipes, I have added a pat of butter to the healthy olive oil. It is so small in calories and fat for the whole dish and adds such a nice flavor that I felt it was worth it. After all, if the food doesn't taste good, how long will you and your family eat it?

Take all the advice and cancer fighting foods listed in the previous chapters and have fun. Learn to cook all your meals with fresh foods that taste great. You will find that your taste will change and your family will be asking for the food that will make you healthy.

Vitamin D and Dogs

When diagnosed with cancer, I started to wonder, as most people with life threatening diseases do, 'Why?' Did I do something to make this disease happen? Is there something that I could have done to prevent cancer from happening? I knew some facts without doing any research. I had smoked cigarettes for 20 years, but I had quit smoking 11 years ago. I was proud of the fact that I was finally able to quit. It took numerous tries, and the help of the patch, but I was proud that I was finally a non-smoker. I didn't think that something I had stopped so many years before could have caused this particular cancer. That is something I will never know for sure.

For 18 years, I had lived in a house with an electric tower in the field behind it. Did that contribute to the cancer? Again, I would never know. I had grown up in the section of New Jersey that the natives called 'cancer alley.' It was called this because of all the pollution caused by the numerous factories and oil refineries located in the area. Did my environment cause the cancer? There was no way to know for sure.

After a time, I gave up trying to figure out why I got cancer. It is a useless indulgence. The important question to ask and find the answer to is how I can keep the cancer from coming back? After all my treatments, surgery, chemotherapy, and radiation, I considered myself cancer-free. The question I needed to ask now is how I was going to stay cancer-free? Some of those answers would surprise me.

My husband loves to tease me about the animals in my life. I have two dogs and 21 Nigerian dwarf goats that I breed each year on my Jersey farm. I started out with nothing but joy while trying to create the farm of our dreams. My husband and I always wanted a farm. It wasn't until the children were almost grown that we made the break from our suburban development and plunged headlong into farming. I started farming with little Nigerian Dwarf goats. I just fell in love with these affectionate creatures. I looked up things on line and found that goats were the easiest animals to care for. With no knowledge, I went to a farm in a neighboring town and purchased three goats. They were all very sick animals and to my sorrow and dismay, they all died within a week.

The sorrow I felt was a catalyst. I went on a 'crusade' to learn all about goats and the diseases that hurt them. I learned about the food that would make them healthy and the plants that would cause them harm. I learned about the vaccinations that would protect them from common goat diseases. I studied the different types of goats and picked the type of goat that would be best for me. In other words, I learned everything I needed to know to keep my little goats healthy and happy. I got a dog - a Labrador retriever - to keep me company on the farm. I purchased chickens to raise and have fresh organic eggs.

I did hours of research to learn what I needed to do to make every little creature on my farm healthy and well. It seems a shame that I never did that for myself. I never took the time to learn what would keep me healthy until my health deteriorated into cancer.

I started to research not only about what makes a person get cancer, but also what keeps a person from getting cancer. The results I found were eye opening. Many of the things that seem to prevent cancer are just common sense. They are lifestyle changes that also prevent other common diseases such as heart disease and high blood pressure. I have already told you how food plays a vital role in preventing cancer. Three other important components may also play a part in a healthy life: exercise, pets, and vitamin D.

My husband has been teasing me for years because of an article he read in a magazine in some unknown waiting room. The article said that many women who are suffering from 'empty-nest syndrome' often buy pets to replace the children. I argued with him and denied it, but had to admit that I got Gracie, my female yellow Labrador, when my daughter took a job and moved to Washington DC. I got Duke, my little Texas Heeler puppy when my son took a job that meant he would not be living at home for six months. Both of my children have grown. My daughter married and my son has a home by the shore. I still have my two dogs. It turns out; however, that having my little pets is a very good thing. Research shows that having pets to love increases the chance of surviving cancer.

All over the world, in the medical and scientific communities, animal shelters and "average Joe's" are all clearly seeing the health benefits from being a pet owner. The Australian Veterinary Association (AVA) states it, "recognizes the importance of the human-animal bond and promotes the benefits of pets to the community." From infants to seniors, the advantages of having an animal companion are numerable.

Researcher James E. Gern, MD, a pediatrician at the University of Wisconsin-Madison said that, a growing number of studies have suggested kids growing up in a home with "furred animals," whether it's a pet cat, dog, or on a farm exposed to large animals have less risk of allergies and asthma.

In his recent study, Gern analyzed the blood of babies immediately after birth and one year later. He found if a dog lived in the home, the infants were less likely (19 % vs. 33 %) to show evidence of pet allergies. They also were less likely to have eczema, a common skin condition causing itching and red patches to appear. In addition, the infants had higher levels of some immune system chemicals, which is a sign that a stronger immune system is being activated.

Autistic children who have pets have been shown to have more pro-social behavior and children in general have a higher self-esteem if there is a pet of any kind in the family. Pets aid in physical activity, teach responsibility and help with emotional growth. Many children are guided by the routine a pet requires, have their first taste of being accountable for another being and learn the importance of sometimes needing to put others before their own wants and desires.

Seniors have been shown to require less medical attention when they are pet owners, which in turn mean less medical costs.

Depression and loneliness is greatly diminished, as well as stress and anxiety; leading to (in some cases) a sense of usefulness and responsibility that is restored. Especially with dog owners, partial stress reduction is due to feeling safer with a "natural alarm."[10]

Pets reduce stress by offering entertainment and distraction from pain and illness. Loving animals brings out a nurturing nature that that we can't always get from people. Maybe it is because animals love us so unconditionally. I only know that each morning, I can't lay around in bed feeling sorry for myself, not when my dogs arise with such joy to start a new day. They can't wait to eat and run outside. They naturally know that each day is a gift. Their joy reminds me each morning that the day is a gift from God. I will not waste it in self-pity or the self-indulgence of depression.

Elizabeth Scott, MS further reports that pets — especially dogs and cats — carry so many benefits, and preventing loneliness is one of them. Rescuing a pet combines the benefits of altruism and companionship, and leaves you with several loneliness-fighters. It can connect you with other people — walking a dog opens you up to a community of other dog-walkers, and a cute dog on a leash tends to be a people magnet. Additionally, pets provide unconditional love, which can be a great salve for loneliness.[11]

My favorite time of the year used to be the cool and crisp autumn. Now that I have the farm, it is the windy and warming spring because the goats 'freshen' in the spring. That means they have babies. They produce triplets and twins of small-multicolored kids. Each day is a surprise as I check the goat pen for the newborns. Holding them and loving them increases my joy. However, it even does more, according to the research compiled by Elisabeth Scott, MS in her newsletter. Research shows that the areas of the brain that deal with social exclusion are the same areas that process physical pain, adding a scientific explanation to the oft-romanticized experience of a "broken heart." One study found that lonely people showed more depressive symptoms, and that lonely and depressed people alike tended to experience less "togetherness" in social interactions. Research has also found that depression and loneliness can feed off of each other, each perpetuating the other. Several studies have linked emotional stress with depressed immunity. Other research links loneliness and depression with poorer health and well-being. That means that people who are experiencing loneliness are susceptible to a variety of health issues.[12]

I already had the pets to bring joy into my life. Now may be the time for you to consider getting a puppy or a kitten. Maybe you always wanted one. I believe a pet can help you heal both physically and mentally. They can replace some of the joy that the cancer may have stolen.

I was never one for formal exercise. In my thirties, I did buy some of the popular exercise tapes. Unfortunately, I watched them as I sat and ate my snacks after work. My life, as the life of most women, revolved around food, not exercise. I planned meals, I shopped for the groceries, and I cooked the comfort food that my mother cooked. Food that made you feel good temporarily, but did little to nourish your body. The meals I cooked were carbohydrate and fat rich, hardly conducive to a walk after dinner. When I did my research, I found that exercise would not only make me lose the excess weight, it would greatly lower the chance that the cancer would reoccur.

Of course, when I decided to give exercise a try, I did what most do. I went overboard and joined a gym. I had to drive for a half an hour back and forth to that gym, but in my enthusiasm, I figured the drive was no problem. I decided to make it to the gym every day. I was in such bad shape from years of sedentary living that it was impossible for me to do the machines. I actually got 'stuck' in a reclining bike during my opening tour of the gym.

My personal trainer quickly changed the exercise regiment he had been planning after that embarrassing episode. He recommended water resistive exercise only. There I was each day, the youngest (and may I say, heaviest) woman in the pool. I jumped around each morning with all the 80 year old women holding their foam 'noodles.' I stayed after class, while all the elderly women soaked in the hot tub, to swim around the pool in laps.

The first two weeks, I went daily, ignoring the fatigue, the muscle aches, and the fact that the rest of my life was falling apart. The third week, I made it to the gym three times. After all, I did have to clean my house, run the farm, and write. By the fourth week, I was showing up twice a week, with an attitude about how this 'exercise' thing was eating up all my energy. By the end of the first month, I was lucky if I was making the gym once a week. Within a few months, I never went back. I was lucky that the gym I joined was nice enough to let me out of the contract. I knew that I was not the type of person to hit the gym each day, or even the three times a week, which is needed for even the smallest result. So, the gym route was not for me.

I quickly discovered that I was not going to do any special exercise that didn't fit into my lifestyle. I knew I would have to find an exercise that I could do at home or just walk out my door and do. But what? I was no more prone to do an exercise tape consistently then I was to go to the gym. I knew that I had to find an exercise that I would do that did not require too many concessions. In other words, it had to have more of a purpose than exercise alone. It had to have some other benefits.

Right around this time, my husband got on a Vitamin D kick. He has always loved the summer sun. Perhaps it is because he works underground as a 'sandhog' or miner in the tunnels of New York. He followed his grandfather and father in this career. In the winter, he would be underground before the sun rose, and arrive above ground after it had set. In the summer, with the longer days, he found joy in the light and warmth of the sun. I always teased him about it, saying that he worshipped the sun like the ancient Egyptians. He countered that 'Ra' was good. One day, during one of the local news programs, it was announced that researchers were becoming convinced that Vitamin D from the sun was proving to be helpful in fighting breast cancer. This supported his love of 'Ra'. He couldn't wait to tell me that his love of the sun was well justified.

I did research to confirm his news and found out that it was true. The work was done by scientists at the University of Toronto. Lead researcher Pamela Goodwin, MD. She is a professor of medicine at the University of Toronto and a senior investigator at the Samuel Lunenfeld Research Institute of Toronto's Mount Sinai Hospital

Goodwin and her colleagues measured vitamin D levels in the blood of 512 newly diagnosed breast cancer patients (95% of them white) and tracked the progress of their disease over an average of about 12 years. About 38% of the women had vitamin D levels low enough to be considered "deficient" and 39% had levels that were "insufficient." Just 24% of the women in the study had "adequate" vitamin D levels.

Women with the lowest levels of vitamin D (deficient) had nearly double the risk of their disease progressing, and a 73% greater risk of death compared to women with adequate vitamin D. The findings were statistically significant, and were not affected by factors including age, weight, tumor stage or tumor grade.[13]

Calcitrol, the active form of vitamin D, has been found to induce a tumor suppressing protein that can inhibit the growth of breast cancer cells, according to a study by researcher Sylvia Chistakos, Ph.D., of the UMDNJ-New Jersey Medical School.

Chistakos, a professor of biochemistry, has published extensively on the multiple roles of vitamin D, including inhibition of the growth of malignant cells found in breast cancer. Her current findings on the vitamin D induced protein that inhibits breast cancer growth are published in a recent issue of The Journal of Biological Chemistry.

Previous research had determined that increased serum levels of vitamin D are associated with an improved diagnosis in patients with breast cancer. Prior to the current study, little was known about the factors that determine the effect of calcitrol on inhibiting breast cancer growth, she said.

During the study, Christakos and co-author Puneet Dhawan, Ph.D., examined the protein involved in the action that can reduce the growth of vitamin D in breast cancer cells. "These results provide an important process in which the active form of vitamin D may work to reduce growth of breast cancer cells," said Christakos. "These studies provide a basis for the design of new anti-cancer agents that can target the protein as a candidate for breast cancer treatment."[14]

Vitamin D is a found in some foods naturally. It is found in fish like salmon and sardines. Manufacturers put it in milk and cereal. It is even put in orange juice now. However the most prominent and natural source of Vitamin D is the sun. Yet there is still a dilemma. Too much sun can damage the skin and even cause skin cancer. That is no small thing to a person prone to cancer. Vitamin D can be taken in supplements, but the experts are divided on what the most effective and yet safe dose is right. Too much of this vitamin can have adverse effects such as nausea, poor appetite, constipation and even too much calcium in the bloodstream. Too much calcium can cause heart abnormalities and kidney problems.

Since my new diet had fatty fish and milk as a good source of vitamin D, I didn't want to take a supplement that might give me too much. I always prefer to get things I need from a natural source. I believe that scientists know so little about what makes the human body or the wonderful world we live in work. However, the God who created this world does and I believe that He created it to give us, his children, the best chance for health and happiness. He created the sun. Why would he create something to harm us? Evidence shows that just fifteen minutes a day in the bright sunlight can give a person all the Vitamin D they need. It was an easy choice for me. I would try to spend at least 15 minutes a day outside. I would absorb all the vitamin D that God wanted to shine on me with no risk of an overdose.

It was then that I had an epiphany, or what some may call a 'light bulb' moment. I needed to be with my dogs, I needed to get some sunshine, and I needed some exercise. What could be easier then to take my little furry friends for a walk each day? It was a slam-dunk decision. Since I had two dogs, I would take one in the morning and one in the evening. I had to start off easy, not being in the best of shape. I started with 15 minute walks and slowly increased the distance and time of my walks every few weeks.

I didn't push myself too hard. I didn't want my walking to be like my gym experience. I wanted to enjoy it, and have it become a part of my life. It turned out to be the perfect exercise for me. My dogs loved it. Each dog relished spending alone time with me and I enjoyed giving them such happiness. I found that my spirits were lifted as I absorbed the sunshine and vitamin D, got fresh air, listened to the birds sing, and enjoyed being outside in nature.

I did some research on walking as an exercise and found that it is known to have numerous benefits. In the Women's Health Initiative study, women who did the equivalent of two hours a week of brisk walking dropped their risk of breast cancer by 18 percent. In the Nurse's Health Study, breast cancer patients who walked from three to five hours a week were half as likely to die from the disease as those who didn't walk. Scientists are planning a clinical trial to test a moderate-intensity physical activity program for breast cancer survivors. Some studies have suggested that moderate exercise might help prevent stomach cancer, endometrial cancer and prostate cancer, but researchers say more research is needed. Why physical activity helps fight or prevent cancer isn't clear, but the key might be in the way physical activity affects hormones or the immune system.[15]

Wow, what a great finding this was to me. I am not the athletic type and trying to do at 50, workouts that I didn't do in my twenties was very depressing. To be honest, even walking was difficult for me at first. I had arthritis from a severe case of Lyme disease and had to walk slowly. It was okay because the more I walked, the easier it became. At first, I did a short, slow walk that didn't leave me in pain or discomfort. As my muscles grew stronger, I found myself walking a little faster and for a longer time each week. It was almost unconscious. I didn't push myself. I didn't want to make walking a chore that would end up like my failed gym experiment. I wanted this exercise to be a pleasure, something that I looked forward to and did for my own pleasure.

In order to do that I had to work on more than my leg muscles, I had to work on the muscle between my ears. I had to change my way of thinking. Just like the positive affirmation of thanking God for my healing each day, I had to find a positive about my choice of exercise. I had to leave behind the past and all the negatives I had about exercise and create a new way of thinking. I had to find my positive. Each day, I would tell myself at any given moment that I couldn't wait to take my walk. I told myself that I loved to walk, and no one was going to talk me out of it. I started to think of my walk as a reward that I gave myself. I told myself that I deserved to have my walk each day.

I convinced myself that walking was my highest pleasure in life. What's funny is that before too long walking was my greatest pleasure. Each morning and evening, I would round out my day with my walk. It became a true delight for me. When I found myself stressed, I stopped reaching for a treat, and found myself reaching for the dog leash. I kept my walks faithfully. I rewarded myself the first month with a new pair of walking shoes. The next month I purchased a pedometer. Walking was fun. I felt stronger. My dogs were happier. It was wonderful.

It was more than wonderful, it was a lifesaver. In May of 2005, the Journal of the American Medical Association published a study that said exactly that. The study said that breast cancer patients who walk briskly for three to five hours a week reduce their risk of dying from the disease by up to 50 percent. Dr Wendy Chen, a member of the team from Brigham and Women's Hospital that conducted the study, said there was a clear-cut explanation for the improvement from exercise.

She said, "In randomized studies, women who exercise have lower estrogen levels and reduced concentrations of hormones that have been shown to increase breast cancer survival. Women who were thinner also do have lower estrogen levels, and the benefits of exercise were greater in women with hormone-sensitive tumors."

For women who walked one to 2.9 hours a week, the risk of death was 20 percent lower than for those who walked less than one hour or did no exercise. For those who walked three to five hours a week the risk was 50 percent lower.[16]

After learning this, it all became a no brainer. I strapped on my walking shoes, leashed up the dog, and walked twice a day. So get up, buy that puppy and walk in the sunshine. Life is a gift from God and 50 percent are better odds that you get with most treatments.

Gratitude

We've all heard the example given to explain the difference between an optimist and a pessimist. They both look at a glass half filled with water and the optimist sees the glass as half full, while the pessimist sees the glass as half empty. Let's hope, if you have been diagnosed with cancer, that you have at least reached the optimist level. Always looking at things negatively is very detrimental to a cancer patient. However, even being an optimist is not enough during trials like this. You have to have gratitude.

What is gratitude? It is a virtue that goes much deeper then optimism. It is so deep that it has to spring outwardly from the spirit. The very core of the person, their very spirit must live in gratitude. This virtue can't be conjured up, nor can the person who desires it, create it. Gratitude is pure grace. It comes from a humble spirit. It is the profound sense of life as gift. In fact, it is the knowledge that everything in life is pure gift.

The grateful person looks at the glass half-full of water and sees the Creator of the Universe as he touched the world with His Word and fashioned flowing steams and roaring rapids. This blessed person sees the beautiful glass that the talent of someone unknown created. The grateful person sees the water sparkling in the hand of someone who offers it because of the generous spirit of the giver. In that simple glass of water they feel the love of the world as it comes together to fill the need they have at this very moment. Wow! No wonder they are filled with such joy. That is the outward sign. Only the truly grateful can have joy.

For the most part, we are a mixed bag. We are happy for some things and feel cheated about others. We may be happy to have a nice home, but annoyed when we have to clean it. We may be grateful to have a nice car but irate about the gas prices. This is not true gratitude. The world teaches us to look for happiness in material things. Material things make us happy for a short time, but the feeling never lasts. That is because happiness is not joy. Happiness is an emotion that depends on outside things. If it is sunny on the day we planned a picnic, we are happy. If it rains, we are not. Happiness is an emotion. Joy is a state. Joy cannot be destroyed by outside circumstances. It is created in the Spirit. I believe it is a gift given by our Creator.

That is why finding happiness from outside conditions never lasts. Looking for happiness in the material things of the world does not work. That new car will grow old and begin to rust. The latest hot invention will be replaced with new technology and be obsolete before you know it. The things of this world cannot bring you joy, because they are temporary. They can only give us joy if we acknowledge them as gifts given by an Eternal Provider. The first step of course is in acknowledging a Creator - a loving Creator who can never destroy what He has created. He can only transform his creation into something even better. He did not destroy the water at the wedding feast of Cana. Listen carefully. He did not replace the water with the wine. He transformed the water into wine. In this small example, the entire nature of our Creator is shown. He destroys nothing, but transforms everything. We have to be humble to see it.

Humility is not low self-esteem. If anything, it is the opposite. We see ourselves as created especially in the love of God. He planned us before time began. We are so important to him that he picked the time and place of our birth. This Loving Creator picked out our hair and the color of our eyes. We are here because He loves us and we should always remember that our stay here is temporary. Life on earth is a gift. This life on earth is not meant to be permanent.

We will not bring any of the temporary things of this world with us when we are transformed to the next. We should enjoy them while we are here, however, our happiness does not lie in the material, but in the one who provides these things. The first step to joy is in asking for the gift of humility. We have Someone in charge and this Someone loves us and has given us this life as a gift for learning. Are we grateful or are we too busy to notice the gifts given each day?

When I was first diagnosed with cancer, I feared that my life was ending. I thought about the things I had accomplished and realized how little my accomplishments were. I looked at the things that I owned and wondered what would happen to all my trinkets and treasures. My unmarried uncle had died just the year before. I remember going up to his home in Jersey City with my mother to take care of the arrangements. His home was full of the remnants of his life. A coin collection, magazines he had kept in piles around his bed. His nightstand held his glasses and his watch, which he had left behind on his hurried trip to the hospital. In his basement were trunks full of varied papers and records he had collected over the years. We took some mementos and the rest were tossed in the garbage. His home sold within a month. And so his life was left without a trace of the material. According to the material world, nothing was left to make a mark, a life had ended and there were no great legacies left to remind the world that he had even been here.

He had left something behind - memories of birthday cards for birthdays never forgotten, visits to the train station and walks home as he held my hand for dinner with my mother. Bags of penny candy that he brought as we strolled by the local store. I remembered hot tomato soup in cracked ceramic mugs with bits of Ritz crackers floating on top. As a child, this gift of lunch was more precious than gold.

I looked around at my own treasures, a collection of angel statues and my most beloved all-clad pots and pans. When I died, would any of these things matter? No, someone would clean up the remnants of my life. What I treasured so would be given away or even thrown away without a thought. I looked at the people in my life; they were the only treasures that mattered. Was I grateful for the gift of the people that blessed my days here on earth? Did I appreciate a loving husband who could always make me laugh? I had two healthy children. God had filled my life with wonderful siblings and friends. Had I really ever thought to be grateful for them? Did I even realize that they were pure gift? I don't think I ever thought of them that way. I was starting to realize how much of a gift these people were. In the end, they would be the only testimony of my life.

During my chemotherapy I made a few friends. There were two in particular who spent the long hours of chemotherapy with me as we sat together each Wednesday. Joann and Terry had breast cancer like me but they were Stage Four. Stage Four is incurable. Each of these women was receiving chemo to extend life, not to sustain it. As Joann and Terry told me when we first met, they were terminal.

Terry's breast cancer had spread to her bones and liver. Joann's cancer had metastasized to her lungs and was now growing in her brain and causing her to go blind. These women became good friends and I enjoyed both of them but they were very different and that difference was profound.

Terry had a good sense of humor but she had a defeated spirit. She felt that life had dealt her a raw deal. She was only middle-aged and didn't think it was fair that her life was to be taken away prematurely. Terry was bitter. In her bitterness, she snapped at her husband. She complained about the food being served and the lack of attention she felt the nurses were giving her. She did it with humor. However, the humor was negative.

As time marched on and her body started to show signs of failing, her negative feelings and humor took on a deeply hurtful and sarcastic quality. She was angry and she took it out on those around her. She felt that life had cheated her and in her negativity, she started to announce that she was 'terminal' with regularity. She was never nasty to Joann and me. I guess she thought that we were in the same boat as her. I remember one Wednesday afternoon, Terry told someone that she was terminal for the third time, and Joann finally addressed her behavior.

Joann said, "We are all terminal, none of us are getting out of here alive!"

It was a simple statement and Terry took it as a joke, but it struck me right between the eyes. All of us are terminal and only God knows when we are coming home to Him. The very proof of that was Joann.

Joann was, without a doubt, the most positive and uplifting person I have ever met. Her joy was infectious. Remember what I said previously about joy belonging to the grateful. I learned that from Joann. She was always smiling. She praised the nurses for their care and they flocked around her for her blessings. She thanked everyone for the sandwiches the volunteers brought and made each week an adventure by trying something new.

She talked with love about her family. She told funny stories about her friends and her pets. Joann was full of gratitude for even the smallest things in life. No one could be sad around Joann. She was deeply religious and talked about all the blessings God had given her. The doctors thought that she would be blind already, but Joann knew better. She said that she had prayed to God not to let her go blind from her cancer, because she loved to read her Bible. I am sure she prayed for a healing but she never talked about it. Joann never complained at all.

Both of these women were terminal with about the same prognosis. Within a few months, I sadly learned that Terry had died. Joann however was home and doing well, at least according to her emails. She emailed me daily. Even her emails were full of joy and gratitude to God for all the little things in life. I am sure she had trials, but she never talked of them. I am sure she had pain, but she only cared about your pain. She spread joy wherever she was and she shared that joy with me. It was a privilege to know her.

Joann passed away two years after our chemo sessions. She never lost her sight and died while reading her Bible. In those two short years that she lived with her cancer, she did more to touch people with love then most people do in a lifetime. She had joy, because she was grateful for each day. I believe that she lived longer because she was so grateful. She wasn't afraid because she knew the well-kept secret. We are all terminal in this life. We are eternal in the next.

Prayer

The Word of God, the Bible, is full of the promises of God for His people. One of the promises is that if we ask, He will answer. In the Old Testament, Psalm 103 says, "Bless the Lord, O my soul... and forget none of His benefits; Who forgives all thine iniquities; Who heals all thy diseases...." [17]

God promises healing. He doesn't promise what kind of healing it will be. I have been a part of a healing prayer ministry in my parish for 18 years. Over the years, I have seen many miracles of physical healing. I cannot explain why one person is healed physically and others remain ill. After all these years, I know better than to try to explain God's work. I can only say that God always heals. The healing may be physical, but in God's eyes, it is more important to heal us spiritually. I think it is because He can see the whole picture. We are eternal beings and this lifetime of suffering is just a moment in eternity.

I have seen God heal emotionally. Often He takes away the depression, sorrow, anger, or bitterness, which accompanies illness. I have seen prayer heal marriages and relationships between parents and children. I have to believe that if we come before the Father as children, He hears our prayers.

My favorite verse in the entire Bible is from Matthew 7:7: "Ask and it shall be given you; seek and ye shall find; knock, and it shall be opened unto you; for every one that asks receives; and he that seeks finds and to him that knocks it shall be opened." [18] That is quite a promise, and it took me the better part of a lifetime to believe it.

As a child, I was taught from my Baltimore Catechism that prayer was 'the lifting of my mind and heart to God.' That definition still holds true. Whenever a person thinks about God, lifting your thoughts from the mundane to the supernatural, you have praised God just by acknowledging Him. However, there are many types of prayer and our circumstances often dictate the type of prayer we use.

The simplest type of prayer is the cry to God in a moment of fear or worry. "Jesus, help me!" may be the most powerful prayer of all when your car is skidding on an icy road, or your children have not arrived home despite their curfew. It is a cry of the heart in a time of danger. I sometimes think it is the purest prayer for it has no forethought and is simply a cry from a child to his Father. A cry of complete trust that the Father can make what is wrong, right again.

As children, we are all taught formal prayer, prayer written by someone else. It is often wrapped in the tradition of whatever denomination or church in which we are raised.

Most Christians know the 'Lord's Prayer.' It is a prayer given to us by Jesus when He was asked how we should pray. It is a deeply meaningful prayer that covers all of our needs. I think it is a prayer that says it all. It is a shame that over the years, as we recite our prayers, they often lose the meaning. We learn to pray without truly feeling the meaning of the words we are saying. We talk at God, not with Him.

I prefer a deeper, meditative prayer during which we carry on a conversation with God. We learn to listen in the silence of our heart for His direction, love, and will. I explain this type of prayer in more detail in the following chapters. Here I want to talk about the power of healing prayer.

"Judaism, Christianity, Islam, Buddhism—every religion believes in prayer for healing," said Paul Parker, a professor of theology and religion at Elmhurst College outside Chicago. "Some call it prayer some call it cleansing the mind. The words or posture may vary. However, in times of illness, all religions look toward their source of authority.[19]

Many people come for prayer for the first time when they become ill. They feel unable to pray for themselves, even unworthy to pray. Somehow, they think that the prayers of those who have been attending church are 'better.' They feel God would not listen to them because they think of themselves as sinners. What they fail to understand is that we are all sinners, and we all fall short.

Often people compare themselves to people they see in church - people they assume are holy. We cannot read another person's heart, only God can. In Matthew 9:12, Jesus says "Those who are well do not need a physician, but the sick do." When our body is sick we do not hesitate to go to the doctor, even if we haven't see him in a few years. When our spirit and soul are sick, we should not hesitate to seek out the Divine Physician.

I think it is important for me to go to church, because when I didn't, I lost my way. Church is what I need to stay centered and focused on God. However, being in church does not make me a Christian any more than my being in the barn makes me a horse. My relationship with God is based on my prayer relationship with him. Do I turn to Him each day and try to discern His Will? That is what builds a lifetime of faith.

Besides, we are taught never to compare ourselves to others. Only God can see the truth in someone's heart. Only God can know how we treat others and if we walk with Him each day. Comparing ourselves to others is a mistake that can only lead to false ideas and envy. We should only compare ourselves to Jesus. In a comparison with Jesus, we all fall short. Are we showing His mercy and love? He is the guide we should use. His love is what we should aim for. Pride cannot enter this similarity, because His holiness is something we can never attain.

Still, the Bible instructs the sick to come to the elders of the church that they may lay hands on them and pray for healing. I believe the humility and faith it takes to walk up the aisle of the church and ask for prayer is the point. God sees the person who seeks before they ever reach the prayer team. He honors the prayer in their heart.

Scientists have been studying the value of prayer in healing recently. Many think that it is impossible to study the effects of prayer. They think that the attempt is like trying to put God in a box and measure Him. Perhaps, it is, but it is an interesting proposal. The answers the scientists receive seem to depend greatly on what the study measures.

It is hard to gauge the power of prayer, because of other variables in the believer's life. Many studies done over the years indicate that the devout tend to be healthier. However, the reasons remain far from clear. Healthy people may be more likely to join churches. The pious may lead more wholesome lifestyles. Churches, synagogues, and mosques may help people take better care of themselves. The quiet meditation and incantations of praying, or the comfort of being prayed for, appears to lower blood pressure, reduce stress hormones, slow the heart rate and have other potentially beneficial effects.[20]

It is under this concept that the scientists believe that religion and the prayer it generates may keep believers healthy. However, I think that they have missed the main point. If God created us, He surely knows how the body He created works. He knows the benefit of meditation and prayer. Knowing that having a relationship with Him is the healthiest way to live, He teaches us to pray and reach out in faith. Those who do are measurably healthier.

Scientific studies demonstrate that individuals who participate in organized religion are physically healthier and live longer. For example, they have lower blood pressure and rates of depression, anxiety, substance abuse, and suicide. Organized religion can promote health through a variety of social mechanisms; discouraging unhealthy behaviors such as alcohol and drug use, smoking, and high-risk sex while providing social support and a sense of belonging.[21]

However, it is the same old argument: which came first: the chicken or the egg? Again, which came first: the health or the prayer? It often comes down to the faith of the interpreter. Studies done by skeptics seem to conclude that the health of believers is result of lifestyle, or the power of suggestion to the believing patient. Perhaps that is why these studies often seem inconclusive.

Blind studies have different results. Prayer researcher Jack Stucki has carried out double-blind studies evaluating the effects of distant prayer on the body's electromagnetic fields. In these studies, the electrical activities in both the brain and body surface were measured in subjects in his Colorado Springs laboratory. Nearly 1,000 miles away in California, spiritual groups would either pray or not pray for a subject. The electrical activity measured in the prayed-for subjects was significantly altered compared to controls. [22]

Double blind studies have also been done to study the influence of prayer on the ill. In a controversial study carried out by cardiologist Randolph Byrd (Southern medical Journal, July 1988), nearly 400 heart patients were randomly assigned to either a group that was prayed for by a home prayer group or a control group. This was a methodologically rigorous double-blind study designed to eliminate the psychological placebo effect. In such a study, neither the patient nor doctor knows who is receiving the intervention (i.e. prayer). Patients who received prayer had better health outcomes, including a reduced need for antibiotics and a lower incidence of pulmonary edema. [23]

There are no scientific explanations for the difference displayed. Some studies are taking a step further in trying to understand why distant prayer can influence subjects who don't even know that someone is praying for them.

Quantum physics is developing theories with insights into non-local phenomena such as distant prayer. For example, Bell's theorem, which is supported by experimental evidence, indicates that once subatomic particles have been in contact, they always remain connected. A change in one creates a concurrent change in the other, even if they are a universe apart. Some physicists believe that these non-local events are not just limited to sub-atomic particles but underline everyday events including prayer. To help understand a number of inexplicable phenomena, including non-local events, many physicists believe that a fifth form of energy exists (in addition to gravity, electromagnetic energy, and strong and weak nuclear energy) that operates on different principles.[24] The studies continue, but while interesting, mean little to me. I know the fifth source of power the scientists are seeking... However, it is not the 'fifth' source of power; it is the First and Eternal Source. I don't know much, if anything, about sub-atomic particles or how they change. I do know that prayer always changes things. When my spirit reaches up and touches God's Holy Spirit, my spirit becomes more. God grants my spirit the grace it needs at the time. Sometimes, I am aware of the change and sometimes I am not, but change always occurs. That change is always good and beneficial, often in ways beyond my limited comprehension.

So if you are sick, turn to your faith and pray. Pray for yourself, and have others pray for you both in person and from a distance. Prayer has power. I have seen that power work in others and I have felt the power within myself. I don't need any scientific study to convince me. I rely on the truth of His Word, which in John 15:7 says- "If you remain in me and My words remain in you, ask whatever you wish and it will be given you. This is to my Father's glory, that you bear much fruit, showing yourselves to be My disciples."[25] In the Old Testament, Hosea 6:1 promises, "Come, and let us return unto Jehovah; for He hath torn, and he will heal us; he hath smitten, and he will bind us up."[26]

Meditations

Many Christians and religious shy away from mediation and guided imagery because the very word 'meditation' conjures up images of Eastern gurus bent in odd positions chanting mantra words to a pagan god. This 'opening' up of the mind to the universe is against the principles of Christianity. We do not know what spirit or entity can enter the person in meditation once they open themselves up to anything. Eastern practices of meditation are geared to finding the 'inner self'; in fact, this type of meditation is all about the study of self. This is not a Christian type of search. So many Christians, however, because of this popular image of meditation shun the practice, unaware that for thousands of years, devout Christians have practiced deep forms of meditation as prayer.

The difference between Christian meditation and the more common 'new age' practice is profound. In Christian meditation, we are not just emptying ourselves and waiting on the 'universe' to send something to fill us. We are emptying ourselves of our ego, our control, our selfishness, in order to make room for Jesus. We make room for the Holy Spirit. As John the Baptist states, 'I must decrease, and He must increase.' We are seeking to fill our spirits with Jesus Christ. We are not seeking our inner and very flawed self. We are looking for the Jesus who says that 'the kingdom of God is within us". This form of deep prayer draws us closer to Jesus and teaches us to hear and recognize His voice and His Will. Monks and saints throughout the centuries have practiced many forms of this contemplative prayer.

One of the most popular types of Christian meditation is called Ledio Divina. In this meditation, a verse or word of scripture is read slowly and repeatedly as the reader digests the Word of God. Sitting in a relaxed and quiet setting, the reader asks the Spirit of God to come and teach the meaning of the selected words in the Bible text. Notice the meditation does not call for an "emptying" as in popular meditation. It calls for an infilling of the Holy Spirit.

The verse is repeated in the mind of the believer until the Holy Spirit takes over and draws the person into an insight of personal meaning as the God of the Universe speaks gently to his creation. Often, if the words are of a scene in the gospel, the person feels drawn into the scene to participate in the story. In this way, Jesus can teach the Christian a principle of holy living or a need to grow in a spiritually individual way. It is a most powerful form of prayer and is practiced by thousands of Christians around the world. I personally practice this prayer each morning in order to grow in knowledge of Jesus.

Guided imagery is the practice of inner healing. Christian therapists and others who understand the practice lead the person into the past, to a bitter memory, or a lingering hate. This time, however, Jesus is there with the person. His healing Love teaches the person to let go of the pain. They are to hand the pain to Jesus. When the person hands their pain to Jesus, the pain disappears and the person is then able to forgive the sin committed against them. The chain of anger is broken. The person no longer needs to carry the heavy chain that has burdened them for so long. Jesus has freed them. For as He says, "The Truth shall set you free" and He tells us how, stating that, "He is the truth and the way and the life."

I am not going to be able to explain or teach the ways of Christian meditation here. That would take many volumes and much more knowledge then your humble writer possesses. I would like to teach you the meditations and guided imageries that I used in my process of defeating cancer. The one teaching that I believe the Eastern religions are correct about is the principle that the mind, body, and spirit of a person work together. When our bodies are sick, we need to not only heal the body, but the affected spirit and mind as well. I believe that an infilling of the Spirit of God is the way to truly heal. I cannot tell you in what direction the Holy Spirit will lead you. I can only share my own experiences and teach you how to put yourself in His presence. He is the Healer, Teacher, and Author of Life. This is how I was able to touch Him daily.

These meditations are written from a Christian point of view. However if you are of another faith, you can simply substitute and create a meditation that works with your belief system. For example, if you are Jewish, simply go to the Spirit of the Creator or God as Father in your meditations. Ledio Divina works wonderfully with passages from the Old Testament, especially the promises of the Psalms. If you are not a believer, create your private meditations on what you think of as a Supreme Being.

This is not a time to remain doubtful. Pray for the Gift of Faith. It is the greatest gift you will ever receive and it will help you through this troubled time like nothing else. So many people say to me that since they have rejected God most of their lives, they feel like hypocrites calling out to Him now that they have cancer. Don't be silly. Our God is a God of Mercy. He is waiting to welcome you to His kingdom of faith. If you take just the first step, He will run to meet you.

Meditation begins with relaxation and breathing. This is no surprise; after all, life begins with the 'Breath of God'. To begin a meditation, get in a relaxed and comfortable position. This means sitting in a chair with both feet on the ground. When I began to do my meditation or guided imagery against my cancer, I picked a comfortable loveseat in my living room. My living room is the most peaceful and relaxing room in my home. It is a simple, comfortable room with no television set. It holds a curio cabinet with all my treasured angel statues and a long table under the picture window that displays all the photos of my family and loved ones. Because it faces the east, the picture window offers the colorful sunrise against the pine trees on my land. It has long been a practice of Christians to face the east in the morning, for as the sun rises, it represents the resurrection of Jesus. In ancient times, all the altars of churches were set up in the East so the prayers of the congregations were directed to the East. I felt blessed to have such a spot to do my prayers and meditations. Here are some of the meditations I practiced:

Breathing in the Healing Light of God

Sitting on my loveseat facing my picture window, I place both feet on the ground and both hands separated on my lap. Looking out the window, I ask God to guide me, as I take in the beauty of His new day. Concentrating on my muscles being relaxed, I shift my concentration to my breathing. Rhythmically, I slow my breathing, taking deep breaths. I then breathe deeply into my nose, hold the breath for a few seconds and then exhale slowly through pursed lips. Relaxing further, and closing my eyes, I concentrate on my breathing. If any thoughts or worries enter my mind, I gently push them away until I am focused again on the breathing.

As I continue to breathe, I begin to notice that the air I am inhaling is cool and light. The air I am exhaling is hot and heavy with moisture. I allow myself to notice this with each breath. In my mind, I start calling the inhaled breath 'healing'. I pictured the healing air flowing right to the site of my tumor. As I exhale the heavy, hot air, I picture it laden with cancer cells. As I continue my breathing I inhale 'healing' imagine it touching the cancer, and I exhale the cancer cells. I picture the cancer in my body growing smaller with each expiration. Continue this until you can picture all the cancer exhaled from your body. This is a very powerful image. This meditation can be repeated daily.

If you are a believer, continue to go deeper. Imagine that the Holy Spirit is present and with each breath, you are inhaling His essence. Inhale the Holy Spirit, let Him touch the cancer, and exhale the cancer. Repeat this exercise until you can actually feel the Holy

Spirit removing the cancer.

Now picture the Holy Spirit as a pure white light. Breathe in the light, watch the light as it touches the cancer, painlessly burning the tumor away. Now exhale the loosened cancer cells. Let the Holy Spirit continue to remove the cancer as you inhale His light and watch Him remove the cancer. Breathe the light out as the light carries the cancer away.

The cancer is almost gone now and a powerful thing happens. The white light takes on a golden glow. Now when you breathe deeply, the Holy Spirit's golden light flows in and stays. The golden light fills your whole body. With each breath, the Holy Spirit flows through your arms and your legs. When you exhale, only a small amount now leaves. As you breathe, your entire body is filled with the Holy Spirit. There is no longer any room for illness or disease.

Continue slowly breathing and the golden light can no longer be contained. The light flows from your fingertips and toes. Can you feel the overwhelming peace and healing of the holy light as it overflows and surrounds your body? It is so powerful. You are full and now overflowing with the healing light. Stay here as long as you can. When you slowly come out of your meditation, do not lose the healing light. Know that it is with you all day. At any time of the day, you can close your eyes and feel the healing light of the Holy Spirit flowing within you, destroying any cancer cells, and carrying them out with every expiration. Remember His Healing Light throughout the day as He flows through you bringing you peace and joy.

A Conversation With God

Sit comfortably in your prayer spot. Keep your feet on the ground and your hands separated on your lap. Relax all of your muscles, from head to toe. Concentrate and become aware of your breathing. Breathe slowly in through your nose, hold the breath, exhale slowly out of your nose. Repeat this slowing of your breathing as you concentrate on the breaths. If any stray thoughts pop into your mind, gently push them away and return to an awareness of each breath. Ask God to come into your presence and surround you with His peace and love.

Think about your favorite place. The place you like to go to be alone and at peace. Is it a deserted beach, or a flower garden? Is it a special place from your childhood? It doesn't matter. Pick your favorite place and go there. For the sake of teaching, I will bring you to my favorite place. Once you understand the exercise, please choose your own.

I close my eyes and find myself walking into a pine forest. I see the sun filtered through the branches of the tall pine trees. My feet crunch as they step on the dry and brown carpet of pine needles along my path. I find my favorite spot, just a short distance from the path. Sitting on the fallen log of an ancient pine, I look around. The pines are so tall in this hidden grove; they seem to touch the blue and cloudless sky. I see the clean, clear water of the babbling stream that runs beside this solitary grove. I see a squirrel as it runs up one of the taller pines nearby. He is carrying an acorn in his mouth as he prepares for the coming winter. It is a cool autumn day. I see a red cardinal fly to his mate awaiting him on a high pine branch. They fly away together.

It is so peaceful and quiet here. I close my eyes. Inhaling slowly, I smell the heavy, clean scent of pine. A light breeze carries the fresh smell of the babbling brook nearby. My breaths grow slower and deeper as I enjoy the fresh clean air. I hear the sounds of the brook as shallow water rushes over the smooth worn rocks. I hear the "caw' of ravens as they fly above. I feel such peace here, in my special secret place. I relax with my eyes closed, enjoying the scents and sounds of this my special place. I know I am in a sacred place as I sense the presence of God. I remain here as long as I like.

I hear soft footsteps approaching. Keeping my physical eyes closed, I open my spiritual eyes. My visitor approaches and sits down on a large boulder facing my fallen log. It is God, Himself. He smiles lovingly and I look deeply into His eyes of peace. He takes both of my hands in His as He faces me. I can feel waves of love emanating from His glowing presence. They wash over me. I am no longer afraid, no longer afraid of anything. Looking into his eyes, I ask my question...

He leans closer to me and answers.

The conversation continues for as long as I want it to. When I am done, He smiles and stands. He places His hand on my head and gives me His blessing. Suddenly, I am back in my pine grove alone. The peace I feel is overwhelming. I stay here as long as I need to; thinking about what God has told me. When I am ready, I open my physical eyes and return to my life.

Many of the saints and mystics of ancient Christianity used the method of prayer that I mentioned at the beginning of the chapter, 'Ledio Divina.' It is taking a verse of scripture and meditating deeply upon it. Many mystics found it very enlightening to meditate on the perfect prayer. The perfect prayer is the one that Jesus gave us Himself. We all know it, but repeat it so quickly that we lose the deep meaning of the words. In the next meditation, we will take the prayer in parts. Some of the ancient mystics would meditate on a small part of the prayer for years. If you are not Christian, simply study the method and use a psalm or word of your faith in a similar manner. This is my meditation. Once you see how it is done, please make it your own. God created each of us as unique and special beings. He talks to us as individuals. What he says to me is not what He will say to you.

The Lord's Prayer

Return to your place of prayer, putting your feet on the ground and your hands loosely separated on your lap. Breathe deeply through your nose, hold the breath in for a few seconds, and breathe gently out of your nose. Concentrate on your breaths as you feel your tensions disappear and your muscles relax. If any stray thoughts come, gently push them away and concentrate on your breathing. Pray that you are entering the presence of the Lord and know that you are in his protective light. When you feel you are ready, concentrate on the following words, repeating them over in your mind until you hear the voice of God. Here is my personal meditation on the holy prayer of Jesus.

Our Father,
Reciting these two words repeatedly in my mind, I focus on the word 'our'

Our? Lord who is this 'our'? Show me who 'our' is. Do you mean my family?

I listen for his voice and the Lord answers me, "Who is your family?"

I stay here for a long time deeply in prayer.

By 'our', do you mean just those in my Church?

The Lord answers me, "Who is in my church?"

Again, I stay here for a long time in prayer.

By 'our', do you mean just those of my nationality, my race?

Again, he answers me, "What is nationality? What is race?"

I stay here for a long time.

Lord, are my enemies included? Lord, what about those people who are cruel and war-like, who kill and hurt others? Listening for His answer, I hear:

'Can you see into their hearts? What right do you have to judge?'

This draws me into deep prayer.

Lord, what about sinners, are you their Father also, you know, those who curse your name, or deny your existence?

Are you not a sinner? Do you always turn to Me?

I go deeply into prayer about this.

So, Lord, you are the Father of all men, those who know it and those who are unaware. You are the Father of all the peoples of the earth and if you are my Father and theirs, then they are all my brothers and sisters. It doesn't matter what church they belong to, you are their Father and I am their sister. It doesn't matter what race or nationality they are. You are their Father and I am their sister. It doesn't matter if they are my enemy, sinners, or those who curse your name. You created them. Therefore, You are their Father and I am their sister. I pray a very long time about this.

It is an overpowering thought to know that all men, women, and children on this earth are part of my family, the children of the same Father. When I look at them, do I see my brother? Do I see my sister? Are all those hurting, hungry, poor, and neglected people my own? If not accepted in my heart as my family, am I calling God a liar? Can God give me enough love and forgiveness for all of them?

Lord, the words, 'Our Father', also mean my Father. What does that mean? How are you my Father? What does the word 'Father' mean?

"So many of my children do not know what a father should be. Their earthly Father was a poor example of what a father is. I am not. I am the perfect Father, your Father. First, I am your Creator. I gave you life."

I ponder this in my heart. He created me. He made me what I am. He created my spirit, my soul, and my body. I stay here for a long time. Deep in prayer I realize that He knew he was going to create me before time began. He picked this time and place especially for me. He knew me before I was created for I existed in His mind and heart. This leads me into a very deep prayer, a deep pondering overwhelms me and my spirit stays here in this prayer for days just touching on His personal love for me.

Then I hear His voice: "A father is a protector. I am your Protector."

Are You my protector? Do you watch over me and save me? Lord, show me the times in my life when You protected me from harm. I am drawn into a deep meditative state as the Lord speaks to my heart.

I ask Him 'Lord, what about the times I was harmed? Were you there? Why was I hurt? Why do I have cancer now?

These are deep questions, and the Lord leads me into a conversation that can last for a long time. My mind can only absorb His knowledge a little at a time. I stay in this conversation for as long as I need to, listening to His voice.

Some things I will not know until I reach the other side. I must come to a place of acceptance in these areas. It is really accepting that I am not God. He loves me and does not need to explain everything to me. A parent does not need to explain why they take a knife out of a child's hand. The child is not the parent. The child has to trust enough in the love and protection of the parent to accept that what is happening is for the good. Still, God will answer many questions with patience and love. He will give me what I need to endure, until I return home to him.

I hear His voice as it says, "A Father is a teacher, one who guides a child to maturity."

Do you guide me? Do you know what I am going through? What am I here to learn? Do you talk to me? Do I listen? Do I even ask? I stay in this place for a long time, pondering the nature of God as my teacher.

Are you like a real father, sometimes teaching us by hard lessons? I remember my earthly father taking me out on a raft in the ocean. I was afraid to swim. Suddenly, I was pushed into the water. Afraid to go under, I doggy paddled as my father watched, until I felt confident enough to swim. Swimming actually became one of my favorite activities. However, at first I was angry with my father for pushing me in the water. I forgot that anger when I learned that I could swim. Is it like that with You, Lord? Are we sometimes pushed into a place of fear or pain to learn?

This led me into a long conversation. There is no time limit on conversations with God. They can last as long as they need to, sometimes for weeks or even months. We may even return to a conversation we thought we finished years later as life lessons continue to present themselves to us.

It occurred to me, what does God the Father look like to me?

I have to admit that when I thought of God the Father, I always thought of the conventional painting of His image. I thought of a stern older man, with a long white beard. He was large and sat on a large golden throne. He held a large golden staff in his hand to strike down sinners and the lost. He was able to strike anything (like Sodom and Gomorrah) with lightning bolts of destruction. Wow, what a frightening image of a Father! Let's look at this horrible image of God the Father and let it become what God the Father really is with the following meditation.

Go to your place of prayer. Keeping both feet on the ground and your hands held loosely on your lap, concentrate on your breathing as your muscles relax. Take a deep breath in and hold it for a few seconds, slowly breathe gently out of your month. Repeat until you are completely relaxed. Now picture the face of your image of God the Father and ask yourself is this how he really looks?

Picture the face of a kind and gentle man who is full of love. Replace your old image with the truth. He is kind and loving. He is your creator, your protector, your teacher. Can you see him now? Remember that face; the face He wants you to see. Now, picture the clothing He is wearing. What clothing would go with that face? Let Him show you how He is dressed. Aren't His clothes casual, soft and warm?

Now change that hard throne into a soft easy chair, a big plush, comfortable looking chair that has plenty of room for you. You are His child. Look at Him. He is holding out His arms to you. There is no fear for you know He loves you. Run up to Him and allow Him to scoop you up to His lap. Lay your head on His shoulder. You can just stay silently safe in His arms, or you can talk to Him. You can go here whenever you want to. St Therese, the little flower, went here every day.

Who art in heaven

'Art': what a strange word. It means 'is'. Our Father is in heaven. Where is heaven?

I pray about this for a long time.

Remembering that I was taught that God is everywhere, I hear him say, "Wherever I am, there is heaven."

I pray about this for a long time, in my mind picturing the places where God is easy to see. At first, I see all the beauty of nature. It is easy to picture God here.

Then I see the horrific images of starving and ill children. I picture the carnage of war. I try to see God there, knowing He is everywhere. How can this be?

I pray a long time about this.

After a time, I remember what Jesus once said that 'the kingdom of God is within me'.

I pray about this and I hear the Scripture, 'deep is calling on deep'.

I feel as if the Spirit of God is reaching deep within me, into my inner spirit. I can sense the Spirit of God within me. Is heaven finding the Holy Spirit within me?

After a time, I ask God about the physical heaven the place we go after we die; I ask if it is a real place. He reminds me of the Bible verse, 'I go to prepare a place for you. In my Father's house, there are many mansions. If it were not so would I go to prepare a place for you? And if I go to prepare a place for you will I not return for you?" [27]

I ask God what my mansion in heaven will be like. Deep in prayer, He shows me a white cottage with a thatched roof just like the cottages of ancient Ireland. The cottage is surrounded with beautiful flowers and I sit in the garden surrounded with puppies and baby goats. I actually laugh at the vision that God is showing me. "Yes Lord, you know me well. A giant mansion would never make me happy. You have given me a heaven just for me, a warm home filled with love, flowers and small animals." I notice that the puppies are the dogs I had in this life, the goats the ones I raised on my small farm. "Yes Lord, You are the author of life. All life is eternal. You could never destroy life." I see my family and friends visiting. My husband sits beside me as Jesus Himself visits. This is my heaven.

What is yours?

This is how you meditate. God does talk to you. In our noisy world, we have forgotten how to listen. This is 'Ledio Divina' I don't need to go further. This is what God said to me. He talks to each person's heart differently for He knows the depths of your heart. Take your scripture, psalm, poetry, or questions and go to Him. The peace you will find will heal you. I can't say how God will heal you. It may be physically, or it may be mentally or spiritually. I wish you peace as you travel this new road of the interior spiritual life. It is a bountiful journey.

Peaceful Ponderings

While I was trying to survive my cancer, I joined a women's support group that met once a week. There I met many women who had been told that they would not survive. These women were of all ages and economic classes. They were of different races and religions. For all of their differences, they all had one thing in common. They had courage. These women taught me that being told that you are going to die has a very profound effect on the psyche. We all know that we are going to die someday. We don't like to think about it. Most of us push this thought away, saving it for old age. It is difficult to realize that we will only live for a period and that when we die, the world will go on without us. Most of the women I met had a deep faith in whatever religion they held. Some did not. Ellen was one of those who did not.

Ellen was short and chubby with blonde hair, or at least the wig was blonde. She was actually bald from the chemotherapy. She always had a smile on her face, despite the fact that she was told a year ago that she had Stage Four, incurable cancer. Ellen was Jewish, but parents who were hard-core atheists had raised her, and she considered herself an agnostic. An agnostic is a person who is not sure whether God exists or not. She was open, but had not been convinced either way. She always listened politely when others in the group talked about their faith. She was extremely interested when they talked about the prayers and meditations that gave them comfort.

One day, because of her husband's work schedule, I gave Ellen a ride home from her chemotherapy. She always felt too shaky after the chemo to drive safely. I noticed for the first time that the smile she always wore did not reach her eyes. It was a mask she was wearing to cover the fear she was living in. As we talked on the long drive home, she brought up the subject of meditation. All of the meditations we had talked about at the meetings were of a religious nature. She just couldn't bring herself to do them.

She asked me if I knew of any meditations that were not religious in nature. Stumped, I quickly said yes, I wanted to help her out of this fear. What I didn't tell her was that I would have to go home and pray for one. I told her that I would bring a written meditation to the meeting. She seems so pleased that I knew I had some serious work to do. I prayed and the following is the meditation I was given. I call it an enclosed garden.

An Enclosed Garden

Get in a comfortable sitting position with both feet on the ground. Close your eyes and concentrate on your breathing. Take deep, long breaths through your nose, hold for few seconds, and exhale slowly through pursed lips. Breathe this way repeatedly as you concentrate on each breath. Relax the muscles in your body from top to bottom. If any stray thoughts come, gently push them away as you focus on your breathing.

When you are relaxed, enter the meditation. Picture a dirt road. You are slowly walking down the unpaved road. Can you see the land you are walking through? Think about the land that you are looking at. You are not alone. You are walking with others. Who are they? Are they family or some friends? It is such a mild, sunny day. You are really enjoying your walk, talking to your companions.

As you are walking, you suddenly hear some music. It is faint at first. You have to strain to hear it. However as you walk, the music becomes louder. Now you are able to hear it. It is the most beautiful musical piece you have ever heard. It touches you in such a profound way. Can you hear the music? Stay here until you can. What kind of music is it?

Enthralled by magical notes, you turn to your companions. They are busy talking, walking quickly ahead. That is when you realize that they cannot hear the music. You ask them if they can hear, and they laugh, thinking that you are joking. They continue walking and you go along with them, but as you walk further, the music starts to fade. Stopping, to listen, you see that your companions keep walking. It doesn't bother you. The music is so beautiful. The notes seem to be calling you, as the music penetrates your heart. The urge to follow it is so strong. You have to find the source of the music. Your companions are far ahead now. They don't seem to notice that you are no longer walking with them.

Turning, you walk back down the road following the sweet sounds of the song. You reach a grove of trees and realize that the music seems to be coming from the thicket. Walking off the road, you follow the music through the wooded area. The music is getting louder and clearer, so you know that you are reaching the source.

Suddenly you see a long and winding wall. The wall is made of heavy stones of various sizes. It is so high that you can't see over it. It must have been here for a long time. Ivy is growing on the thick, high wall. The music is so close now. It is coming from behind the wall. You walk along the wall on a little path that follows the length of the wall. There must be an opening. You want to see where to music is coming from.

Walking for a few minutes following along the wall, you realize that you hear other sounds from behind the wall. It is voices. People seem to be laughing and joking as the music continues. Some of the voices sound so familiar.

Finally, you see a gate, a high wooden gate. It is so solid and high you can't see into the area beyond the gate. You look for a latch but there is no latch. You can hear the laughter and the music, as crowds of people seem to be enjoying themselves. Can you hear them? Do any of the voices seem familiar? You can't wait to join them. They seem so happy. However, as you stand before the gate, you know there is no way for you to open it. You will have to knock. Do you?

When you knock, the noise of conversations stop, but the music continues. You can hear someone on the other side approaching the gate. You step back as you hear a heavy metal latch squeaking open. The large ancient gate swings slowly open and you can see the person who opens it smiling at you. Who opened the gate? You know who it is immediately. Peeking in, you see all the people, as they smile at you. You know them all. The person who opened the gate smiles deeply at you. You can talk to them now. Ask them anything you like. Talk as long as you need to.

When you finish talking, you realize that it is not time for you to go inside the garden yet. You have to leave as the gate is closed. As you walk back to find your companions on the road you have to hurry to catch up with them. They welcome you with smiles but continue without asking you where you have been. You can still hear the music of the enclosed garden but it grows fainter as you walk away. You are not concerned. You know you can return to the walled garden whenever you want to. Relax and slowly come out of your meditation. Remember the people you have seen. Reflect on what they have told you, at peace, knowing that you can go back whenever you want.

Ellen loved this meditation. She told me in the coming months that she often did it twice a day. I never asked her what music she heard. I never asked her who opened the gate. It seemed too private. I did notice that the fear seemed to leave her. Now when she smiled, the smile was in her eyes. She eventually left the group because her cancer came out of remission and attacked her vigorously. She was too weak to continue and eventually she died at home with her family and friends around her. I have no doubt, that she walked over the threshold of the gate and entered the garden of peace. I don't really know who opened the gate for Ellen. Hope alone tells me who it was.

Two of the women in our little group were also dying, their cancer held temporarily in check by heavy doses of chemo. They were Christians and the two had become fast friends as they shared a common faith and disease. One was born-again and the other was Orthodox. When Ellen bragged about her new meditation, they begged me to write one for them. After prayer, I knew that nothing I could write would be better than meditating on the prayer called 'The Apostle's Creed.'They loved it.

As far as I know, they are still practicing it today. I eventually left the support group as my schedule changed. I hope it brings you as much peace as it brought them. You do not need to be dying to do this meditation. You do not even need to be ill. Again, go into a comfortable meditative state as spoken of previously and meditate on each line. You can stay on a line for as long as you want. It can be days, or even weeks before you are ready to go to the next line. Remember this is not a race. It is not about going fast or finishing. The longer you stay with a line, the deeper your insight will be and that is what is important.

The Apostle's Creed

I believe in God,

What a powerful statement!   Do you really believe?

Why?

Can you see God in nature?

Can you see God in the people around you? Can you remember times that God saved you?

Can you talk to God? Does He talk to you? Do you listen? What is He saying?

What does your God look like? Is He a kind God? Does He care about what is happening to you? How do you know? Has He helped you in the past? How?

Where do you go to meet Him?

Do you have a special place? What is His voice like? Do you always recognize His voice?

Does He talk to you when you are not at prayer? Can you remember times you suddenly heard His voice and recognized it. What has He said to you?

As you can see, this one little line can lead you into a much deeper relationship with God. Talk to Him about your illness, He is waiting to talk to you. You will be lead into other questions of your own. Your conversation with God will be unique, because you are unique.

The Father,

Is He your father? How do you know? Does He act like a father? Do you act like His child? Can you go to Him for comfort? Can you picture Him holding you as a loving father would hold a child? Or are you afraid of Him? Talk to Him about this, talking as long as you need to. You can come back here as much as you want and talk to Him. Can He teach you that He loves you? Can He teach you not to fear? Talk to Him. Can you stay here until you know that you are His child and that He loves you?

Almighty.

Almighty? What does that mean?

Do you really believe that He is all-powerful? Can He do anything? Is He in charge of everything?

Have you asked him to heal you? Why not? Are you afraid of the answer? Have you talked to Him about the cancer? What about the pain? Are you angry with Him over it? Can you tell Him that you are angry? What does He say?

Can you understand what He is saying? Can you accept it? If not, keep talking.

Have you stopped talking because you are angry? Do you think He is angry? Do you think the illness is a punishment? Do you think that God gave you the cancer? Or did He just allow it? Keep talking.

Can you reach out to Him? Can you turn to Him and accept

that what He allows is the best for you? Keep talking as long as you need to.

This talk should take a long time, and you can return to this talk repeatedly whenever needed. A conversation will change often over the course of your illness. You can spend weeks on one question alone. Let God lead you.

Epilogue: Living with Cancer

A strange thing happened in 2008, four years after I was first diagnosed with cancer. I went for my six-month checkup and was told I was ready to be moved to the survivor group. My first reaction was that it was great news. I was a survivor. I no longer had to think of myself as a cancer patient. I was now officially a cancer survivor. It didn't hit me until the drive home how much this frightened me.

In fact, it terrified me because I had grown used to the safety of being checked every six months by the two doctors who, in my opinion, saved my life. Now, as a survivor, I was no longer going to see my doctors. I was going to be assigned to a nurse practitioner who would oversee my recovery. I was also going to have my mammograms done every year, instead of every six months, just like a person who never had cancer. The whole idea made me nervous. Cancer can grow so much in a year. I was afraid the cancer would come back and no one would know until it was too late.

It was time to move on. I knew that in my mind, but fear wrapped itself around my heart like a snake. I put on a good face. I told everyone how happy I was about being an official survivor. I knew my thoughts were ridiculous, so I wouldn't admit my true feelings, not even to myself. It seemed unreasonable for me to be afraid of having won the hard fought battle against cancer. But you see, that was just it.

I had spent a year with surgeries, chemotherapy, pneumonia, and radiation. I had changed my diet, prayed, walked, and meditated my way through cancer. Being a cancer patient had become my identity. Wow! My life had been on hold. I spent all my time trying to transcend my diagnosis. All my free time was spent Googling the latest research, and shopping for organic food. I didn't just cling to life. I learned to hold on to life with both hands. Now I was told that I won, I had won in my battle over cancer. The problem was my hands were cramped, unable to move, because of holding on so tightly.

I guess you wondered where the story of my son being stuck in the gumball machine fit into the tale of my healing. Well, here it is. I was holding on to life too tightly. It was good to cling to life during my treatment and I have no doubt that my day-to-day efforts helped me to defeat the killer. But now it was time to let go, let go of being a cancer patient.

I have heard of many 'cancer survivors' who go into deep depression when the battle is finally over. Suddenly the side journey of the cancer experience ends and we are to join the main thoroughfare of life again. We think the trouble is that we've forgotten how to walk and where our life was going before the cancer. The real problem is that we are different people now. We cannot go back to our old journey, because we are not the same people. Cancer has changed us. Our outlook on life is different. We know the fragility of life. We know it may end at any time. It is not that we are living in fear. It is that we have overcome the fear of death. The healing has made us different. However, all the people in our life expect us to go back to who we were, to pick up where we left off. That is just not possible.

I was clinging to life with both hands, going through massive changes in my habits and painful treatments with stoic strength. I held on tightly to life. Like my son, stuck in the gumball machine, I finally won the prize, but lost my freedom. I lost the freedom of waking up and not thinking of cancer, or cancer treatments, or even my new friends who had been on the side path with me. The new friends who were all in the battle with cancer, I was leaving them now. Oh, I don't mean that we would not continue to be friends, but the friendship would change. I was no longer fighting the same battle and while I could encourage them in their fight, it would be from the main road. I was off the side path. I was back in the land of the healthy.

The thing about being cured was I didn't know how to let go of being sick, in fact I couldn't let go. If I put down my guard, would the cancer return to fight another day? What new life waited? I was a Christian writer, but I had changed. Could I write the same way as before the cancer? Of course not! My faith had changed. It grew in such a deeply personal way, I didn't know if I could find the words to share it. I learned God and my eternal life with Him was all that mattered. Oh, don't get me wrong, I wanted to live a long life on earth. However, my perspective had changed. Would I be able to convey the deep and loving relationship I had developed with the God who healed? Some things are beyond the written word.

However, that was only part of my problem. I had to let go of cancer. Physically I had defeated cancer, but could I defeat it emotionally and spiritually? Could I let go? Could I pull my hand out of the fear and anxiety and let go?

For the last four years, I had been dancing with death. Now that the music had stopped, could I stop the dance? I watched some of the cancer survivors who went before me. Some of them become so defined by the disease that they became 'professional survivors.' Oh, to the rest of the world it seemed what they were doing was good; they went to every cancer rally, walked or ran for the cure and turned most of their wardrobe to a study of pink. They were raising money for research and that was good, but were they finding the new person they were after the cancer? No, I didn't think they were. They still identified themselves with a disease. Everything they did related to the disease; weekends devoted to arriving at every rally as the sign of hope for the sick. It created great camaraderie and hope for those who were sick, but what about the people who were cured?

I felt that it was time to get off the side path and return to the main road of life. It was the unknown that turned me back. Yes, I was a cancer survivor, but I was a whole lot more than that. Could

I let go? I was holding on to life so hard, and it was all about worry. The biggest fear was that the cancer would return. In the morning, I woke up with the anxiety, and at night I went to bed with the same fear. Yes, I knew I had just lived through a miracle. The fact that I discovered Stage One of a very aggressive type of cancer in my first mammogram couldn't be anything else but a miracle. I had to let go of all the terror of recurrence. The odds were in my favor. It was very unlikely I would have cancer again. The question was would I ever have my life back again?

I was losing the freedom and joy in life. I was holding on to life so tightly that I couldn't enjoy it. I finally had to let go. I let go of the terror. I let go of the cancer survivor identity. I even let go of any sense that I had any control over whether I would live or die. No one has a guarantee. No one has a promise of tomorrow.

What I did have was today. Did I want to spend it waking up and thinking of cancer? Or did I want to wake up to the joy of the morning and the anticipation of a happy day? Did I want to look in the mirror and see a former cancer patient or a woman full of happiness and love? The answer was simple. I had to let go, and let it be. It's so funny now that I think of it. Since I was a teenager, my favorite song is the Beatle's song: "Let it Be." Especially the line, "When I find myself in times of trouble, Mother Mary comes to me. Speaking words of wisdom, Let it be. Let it be.'

Whenever a person hangs on to something tightly they become the slave to whatever that thing is. They do not possess it, it possesses them. My son learned that with a red gumball in a gumball machine. I learned that from cancer. Life is a gift. We should appreciate it. We should enjoy it. We should fight to keep it when the circumstances warrant the fight.

However, when we cling to anything, including life, we are living in fear. My son feared that in letting go, he would lose what he wanted. Instead, the fact that he clung so tightly meant that he didn't enjoy the gumball and he was a prisoner to his greed and fear.

When you let go of the fear of losing this life, you can begin to really live. You are able to experience all of the things you always wanted to. Give up your fear of flying and travel. It is really a fear of death. Give of your fear of heights and experience the joy of the Empire State Building on a star-filled night. Let go of your fear of animals and learn to bond with one of God's special creatures. All of life is about letting go and living. Let go of your fear of death and learn to live. I don't know if the cancer will return or not. It doesn't matter. I have let go of cancer. I have let go of the fear of death.

What does that mean? I never turn down an invitation to spend time with a friend, a pet, my family, or a stranger. I never turn down the chance to travel to a new place, or experience an adventure, or even the chance to try a new cuisine. I have let go of the fears that held me bound and in that freedom, I have met the true joy of living. Let go of the cancer. Let go of being a cancer patient. Let go of being a cancer survivor. Be free to be yourself, the fearless child of a joyful God.

Appendix A: Recipes

Breakfast Recipes

Fruity Oatmeal

Cook steel-cut oatmeal as directed for the amount of servings needed but instead of using water use low fat milk. Add to the mixture ½ teaspoon of ground flax seeds per serving. When the oatmeal is cooked add one small, sliced banana, 1/3 cup of blueberries and one tablespoon of local honey* per serving. Mix well, and serve in bowls.

Tasty Omelet

Ingredients:
Three free-range, organic brown eggs
Pam spray, or teaspoon of olive oil
½ a cup of spinach leaves, chopped
½ a cup of reduced fat feta cheese

Heat a skillet with some oil or spray over medium heat. Beat your three eggs in a bowl and pour into heated skillet. Cook eggs until the edge seems to be cooking. Top with spinach and feta cheese. Loosen one side of the egg with a spatula and flip that side over the other to form an omelet. (Don't worry if it doesn't work, just mix and serve as spinach and feta scrambled eggs, it's not worth the stress) Serve with whole-wheat toast and fruit.

Tasty Breakfast Smoothie (for a day on the run)

In a blender, add one cup of low fat milk and one cup of crushed ice. Add a small banana, 1/3 cup of blueberries or strawberries and a tablespoon of local honey* or some sweetener like Splenda and blend until smooth (Sugar causes inflammation) If you have time add a slice of whole-wheat toast with organic peanut butter and you're ready to run out the door.

*Local honey is made by bees that use the pollen in your area to create the honey. Small doses of this local honey will slowly teach your body to tolerate the pollen in your area. Next time the pollen season arrives, your allergic reaction should be less. Remember less stress allows your body to concentrate on fighting the cancer.

Lunch Recipes

Wilted Cabbage and Mushrooms

Ingredients:
One small head of green or red cabbage or ½ of a large head, roughly chopped
One cup of sliced and cleaned mushrooms, I like to vary the type as each has a different healing power
One teaspoon of crushed flax seeds
One large onion, chopped
1/2 a cup of toasted sesame seeds
Two tablespoons of olive oil
One pat of butter
Teriyaki sauce

Salt and pepper

In a large skillet, heat the olive oil and butter. Add the onions and cook on medium for a minute until soft. Add the mushrooms and cook for a minute. Season with salt and pepper. Add the chopped cabbage and cook over medium heat with the cover on until the cabbage wilts - it is important to keep checking and stirring to prevent burning. Once the cabbage wilts add the sesame seeds and season again with salt and pepper. Add the teriyaki sauce to taste. Turn the heat down to low and if you are a vegetarian add tofu crumbles. If you still eat chicken or turkey, add 1/4 of a pound of precooked and chopped turkey bacon and mix. Serve alone for lunch or as a side dish for dinner.

Oven Roasted Vegetables

I love this recipe. I make this every week and I make a huge amount so that I can have it on hand for a side dish or a lunch. It is packed with nutrients and can be varied as vegetables come and go out of season.

Ingredients:

Preheat the oven to 450 degrees

Into a large roasting pan that has been coated with olive oil, add

One bunch of celery chopped into two-inch pieces

One butternut squash peeled and cut into big chunks

Two large onions peeled and cut into big chunks

Three large yams peeled and cut into chunks

Two packages of mushrooms (two different kinds) washed and put whole into mix

Large bag of fingerling carrots that are peeled and washed

Four large unpeeled white potatoes cut into chunks (do not peel skin)

½ pound of washed, fresh string beans that have the ends snapped off

Lay the vegetables out as evenly as you can on the bottom of the pan and spray with Pam or drizzle with olive oil. Salt and pepper to taste. Add lots of minced garlic (at least two tablespoons) You can add any spices that you have or like. I like fresh or dried basil but have also used chopped rosemary or parsley. Put the pan in the oven for at least a half an hour, stir the vegetables frequently until the vegetables start to caramelize. Remove from the oven and let cool. Place in individual serving containers or bags.

Mock Hamburgers with Sweet Potato Fries

*Ingredients:**
Two large yams or sweet potatoes peeled and cut into fries
Two large Portobello mushroom caps, washed
Pam or olive oil
Montreal steak seasoning
Salt and pepper
Two large whole-wheat buns
Whatever 'fixings' you normally put on your hamburgers

Preheat oven to 450 degrees. Spray a large roasting pan with Pam spray. Lay out your fries in single layer and lay your mushroom cap with the top up. Spray with Pam or sprinkle with olive oil, Salt and pepper to taste. Place in oven for ten minutes. After ten minutes, turn your mushroom caps so the top is down, sprinkle lightly with Montreal steak seasoning. Turn your fries with a spatula and spray everything with Pam. Check oven every five minutes until your fries are caramelized and crispy. Plate your fries, and place the mushroom caps on the buns and prepare with your favorite hamburger fixings. Enjoy!

Dinner Recipes

Pasta Primavera

Ingredients:
One pound of whole-wheat angel hair pasta
One large can of tomato sauce
One large can of tomato paste
Two teaspoons of Italian seasoning
One tablespoon of minced garlic
Two tablespoons of a good olive oil
One tablespoon of local honey*
½ teaspoon of black pepper
One teaspoon of salt
½ pound of fresh broccoli florets
½ pound of fresh cauliflower florets
½ pound of carrots cut in small rings or thin carrot fingerlings

First, start the sauce by placing the olive oil in the bottom of a pot and heat over medium heat. Add the garlic and cook for a minute (do not burn as it will become bitter). Add the can of tomato sauce and the can of paste and stir well. Bring the pot to a boil and then reduce to a simmer. Add the Italian seasoning, spices and honey, then stir, and continue to simmer in an uncovered pot. Cut your vegetables into bite-size portions and add to the simmering sauce. Boil your water and cook your pasta el dente as the package instructs. Drain your pasta and plate, cover your pasta with a ladle of the vegetable red sauce and serve with fresh ground parmesan cheese.

Serving suggestion: Italian garlic bread. Go to a bakery to buy your bread, if you don't have the time to make your own.

Bakery bread is free of preservatives. Even if you must have 'white' bread, get it from a bakery. Slice the bread lengthwise and place on cookie sheet. Heat your oven to 400 degrees. In a small pot heat ½ cup of olive oil with one pat of butter over medium heat. Add two tablespoons of minced garlic and one tablespoon of Italian seasonings. Remove from heat when the butter melts and spoon or brush the mixture over your bread. Sprinkle your bread with parmesan cheese and grated low fat mozzarella cheese. Place in oven and bake for 5-10 minutes just until the cheese melts. Slice into pieces and serve with the Pasta Primavera.

Turkey Meatloaf Dinner with
Sweet Mashed Potatoes and Early Peas

Ingredients:
Two pounds of ground turkey meat
One cup of one-minute oatmeal
One tablespoon of crushed or ground flax seeds
½ cup of chopped onions
½ cup of chopped peppers
½ teaspoon of dried basil
One teaspoon of salt or seasoning salt
½ teaspoon of black pepper
One egg
½ cup of low fat milk
½ cup of ketchup
¼ cup of mustard
One canister of refrigerated crescent rolls
Four large yams
2 tablespoon of butter
One tablespoon of cinnamon or apple pie spice
½ cup low fat milk
Can of early peas

Preheat the oven to 350 degrees. Wash yams and place on oven rack. In a large bowl mix turkey meat, oatmeal, onions, peppers, spices, egg and milk. Mix well with hands until firm (it should feel a little wetter than traditional meatloaf) If it is too wet add more oatmeal until you can form a loaf. Place the loaf in oven ready pan brushed lightly with oil olive or sprayed with Pam. Put in oven for forty five minutes. Mix the ketchup and the mustard in a bowl. Remove the yams from the oven (Make sure they are done by poking with a fork). Remove the turkey meatloaf and pour the ketchup and mustard mixture over it. Open up the crescent rolls and cover the meatloaf with it, Place the meatloaf back in the oven for fifteen more minutes until the crescent cover is golden brown. In the meantime, cut the yams in half and scoop out the soft flesh and place in a bowl. Add the butter and milk and the cinnamon or apple pie spice and mash until the consistency of mashed potatoes

Heat your early peas. Remove the meatloaf from the oven when ready and let sit for five minutes. Slice and serve with mashed yams and peas on the side.

Pecan Crusted Salmon with Whole Wheat Couscous and Sautéed Broccoli

Ingredients:
Two six ounces filets of fresh salmon
One cup of whole pecans
Olive oil
Salt and pepper
One box of whole-wheat couscous
Two large crowns of fresh broccoli
One pat of butter
One tablespoon of minced garlic

½ chopped onion
One teaspoon of ground flax seeds
Two tablespoons of chopped fresh rosemary

Preheat the oven to 400 degrees. Brush an oven-ready pan with olive oil. Place the pecans in the blender and chop into small pieces. Brush the salmon with olive oil and salt and pepper. Sprinkle with the chopped rosemary and crushed pecans and put in oven. While salmon is cooking, make your couscous according to directions

Cut your broccoli crowns into florets. Heat your onion and minced garlic in skillet with tablespoon of olive oil and one pat of butter. Add your broccoli and crush flax seeds and stir constantly while you sauté over medium heat until the broccoli is done but still crisp. The salmon cooks in about twenty to thirty minutes according to cut and size, when you are sure it is done, remove from oven. Plate your broccoli and couscous on each half of the plate, Place your salmon filets on top of the couscous and serve.

Footnotes

1. U.S. Dept. of Health and Human Services, "Mammograms," Office on Women's Health, April 2006, http/www.womenshealth.gov/faq/mammography.htm, {access Oct 15, 2007}

2. Oncology Channel, "Breast Biopsy," Creative Mesh, April 1999, http//www.oncologychannel.com/breastcancer/breastbiopsy/needle.shtml, {access Oct 26, 2007}

3. Oncology Channel, "Breast Biopsy," Creative Mesh, April 1999, http//www.oncologychannel.com/breastcancer/breastbiopsy/needle.shtml, {access Oct 26, 2007}

4. Oncology Channel, "Breast Biopsy," Creative Mesh, April 1999, http//www.oncologychannel.com/breastcancer/breastbiopsy/needle.shtml, {access Oct 26, 2007}

5. New American Bible. (New York: Catholic Book Publishing Co. 1992) 145 John 1:1

6. New American Bible (New York: Catholic Book Publishing Co. 1992) 5 Gn. 2:7

7. Duke University Health system, "White blood cell booster may help cancer patients avoid deadly complications," DukeHealth.org, copyright 2004-2008, www.dukehealth.org/healthlibrary/news/10081?search-highlight=complications

8. Stein, Rob, "Breast Cancer Risk Linked to Red Meat, Study finds," The Washington Post, November 14, 2006, A01.

9. Tally, Steve, "Tomato packs more cancer-fighting punch," Perdue News, June 17, 2002, Http://news.uns.purdue.edu/htm14ever/020617.honda.lycopene. html, accessed June 22, 2008.

10. Boven, Marie, "The Healing Power of Companion Animals," Equine Articles, 14 Nov. 2008, http://ezinearticle/?The-Healing-Power-of-Companion-Animals,1691523

11. Scott, Elizabeth MS, "Loneliness, How to Cope with Loneliness," About.com, Feb 14, 2006, http://stress.about.com/edpsychologicalconditions/a/loneliness.htm.

12. Scott, Elizabeth MS, "Loneliness, How to Cope with

Loneliness," About.com, Feb 14, 2006, http://stress.about.com/ed/psychologicalconditions/a/loneliness.htm.

13. "Study Sees Link Between Vitamin D, Breast Cancer," American Cancer Society News Center, 5/16/2008, http://www.cancer.org/docroot/nws11xstudyseeslinkbetweenvitaminDbreastcancer.asd

14. Chistakos PH.D., Sylvia, "Vitamin D Found to Stimulate a Protein that Inhibits the Growth of Breast Cancer Cell," Science Daily, Feb 5, 2009.

15. Nuzza, Regina, "Walking shows disease-fighting powers, Los Angeles Times. March 12, 2007.

16. Chen MD, Wendy, "Physical Activity and Survival after Breast Cancer Diagnosis," Jama, May 20, 2005

17. New American Bible (New York: Catholic Book Publishing Co. 1992) Proverbs 103

18. New American Bible (New York: Catholic Book Publishing Co. 1992) Matthew 7:7

19. Stein, Rob, "Researchers look at Prayer and Healing," Washington Post, Friday, March 24, 2006

20. Stein, Rob, "Researchers look at Prayer and Healing," Washington Post, Friday, March 24, 2006

21. Koenig, Harold, "Religion is Good for Your Health," 1997

22. Johnston PH.D, Laurence, "The Science of Prayer and Healing," Prayer & Healing, August 9, 2008. http://www.healingtherapies.info/prayerandhealing.htm

23. Stein, Rob, "Researchers look at Prayer and Healing," Washington Post, Friday, March 24, 2006

24. Johnston PH.D, Laurence, "The Science of Prayer and Healing," Prayer & Healing, August 9, 2008. http://www.healingtherapies.info/prayerandhealing.htm

25. New American Bible (New York: Catholic Book Publishing Co. 1992) John 15:7

26. New American Bible (New York: Catholic Book Publishing Co. 1992) Hosea 6:1

27. New American Bible (New York: Catholic Book Publishing Co. 1992) John 14:2-3

About Author
Karen Kelly Boyce

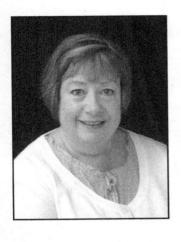

Karen Kelly Boyce was born in Jersey City, NJ. She learned her faith and love of reading at the hands of the Sisters of Mercy. Only a few blocks away from the Barron Library, she spent most of her summer days and weekends lost in the stories and biographies of famous people. The turbulent sixties led her away from her first loves of church, reading, and writing. The only part of her faith that remained was the belief that we were made to help others. That belief led her to graduate as an RN in 1974.

Karen married in 1975, and raised two children. After going through a Life in the Spirit Seminar, she found peace and eternal love in the faith that would sustain her. In 1990, she became very ill and was eventually diagnosed with end stage Lyme Disease and was unable to work as a nurse any more. As a disabled person, Karen's love of reading was rekindled and her love of writing born again.

Karen is also the author of three fiction books - *According to Thy Word, Into the Way of Peace.*, and *Down Right Good.* Karen is available for book talks and signings by calling 732.928.7981 or by email: donegalarizona@yahoo.com.

All books can be purchased on line at :

www.queenofangelsfarm.com or
www.jacksonwritersgroup.com/boyce.html